STOPPING BLOODBORNE HIV

Investigating Unexplained Infections

Adonis & Abbey Publishers Ltd

St James House
13 Kensington Square,
London, W8 5HD
United Kingdom

Website: http://www.adonis-abbey.com
E-mail Address: editor@adonis-abbey.com

Nigeria:
Suites C4 – C6 J-Plus Plaza
Asokoro, Abuja, Nigeria
Tel: +234 (0) 7058078841/08052035034

British Library Cataloguing-in-Publication Data
A catalogue record for this book is available from the British Library

ISBN: 978-1-913976-01-9

Printed and bound in Great Britain

STOPPING BLOODBORNE HIV

Investigating Unexplained Infections

David Gisselquist

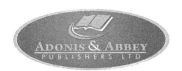

Acknowledgements

This book follows years of informal and formal discussions about bloodborne risks for HIV in Africa and about how to stop or avoid them. During these years, hundreds of non-medical people aware of the risks have shared with me their thoughts about what they can do to protect themselves and their families. I cannot thank them by name, but I hope what I write here accurately reflects their experiences.

I thank Lucy Hancock and Steve Minkin for their encouragement from 1999, when I began to search medical journals for information. Thanks also to people I met through the Safe Injection Global Network, including especially Yvan Hutin, Jules Millogo, and Lone Simonsen, for questions, guidance, and advice.

I thank many co-authors – collaborators and often tutors – who have helped me to assess and present evidence of bloodborne HIV transmission in Africa, including especially John Potterat, Devon Brewer, Stuart Brody, Francois Vachon, and Garance Upham.

Mariette Correa invited me to join with her and Deodatta Gore to research bloodborne risks in India. Out of that research, we three developed a set of recommendations to help people see and avoid bloodborne risks. Thanks to Simon Collery for helping to put those recommendations on a website (bloodbornehiv.com).

I thank John Potterat, Mariette Correa, Joseph Sonnabend, and Simon Collery for reading all or portions of early drafts of this book and for advising on content. Simon Collery helped to prepare the manuscript for publication. Thanks to Jideofor Adibe and his staff at Adonis & Abbey for encouragement and support to bring this book to market. Certainly confusions and errors remain, despite all the good advice I have received. I'll claim those.

Finally, I would like to thank my wife, Carol, for supporting my work on this topic for years and for good advice on arguments and content.

David Gisselquist
October 2020

Table of Contents

List of Tables and Figures vi

Acknowledgements.. iv

Acronyms viii

Chapter One
Purpose and Outline.. 1

Chapter Two
Investigating Unexplained HIV Infections outside Sub-Saharan 13

Chapter Three
Health Experts Advise Africans: Ignore HIV from Health Care 39

Chapter Four
African Governments Accept Unexplained HIV Infections.................................. 59

Chapter Five
Evidence from a Double-barreled Smoking Gun 75

Chapter Six
Rejecting the Myth that Almost All HIV Comes from Sex................................. 79

Chapter Seven
Errors and Delays in Responses to Africa's HIV Epidemics.............................. 97

Annex 1
HIV/AIDS Epidemics in Africa 119

Annex 2
Unethical HIV Research in Africa 129

Index 143

List of Tables and Figures

Table 2.1:   Investigated outbreaks with more than 100 HIV infections 13

Table 2.2:   How many health facilities transmitted HIV, and what did the country's HIV epidemic look like in 2019? 29

Figure 3.1:   Percentages of health facilities with equipment to process instruments for reuse 49

Figure 4.1:   Percentages of self-reported virgin men and women aged 15-24 years who tested HIV-positive in national surveys 60

Figure 4.2:   Percentages of HIV-positive children with HIV-negative mothers from national surveys...60

Table 4.1:   New HIV infections in women during pregnancy and after delivery 62

Figure 6.1:   What do similar HIV sequences say about how many HIV infections come from sex? 82

Figure 6.2:   Percentages of traced adult contacts testing HIV-positive vs. percentages HIV-positive among all adults in the country? 85

Table 6.1:   Estimated rates (% per year) at which women age 15-24 years got HIV from sex, six countries in southern Africa, 2015-17............86

Figure 6.3:   Comparing the estimated rates women aged 15-24 years got HIV from sex vs. the observed rates they got HIV from all risks, 2015-17..87

Figure 6.4:   Slow HIV transmission between couples in seven African countries 89

Figure 6.5:   HIV infections do not concentrate in sexually more active adults 91

Figure 7.1:   Percentages of HIV-positive people in sub-Saharan Africa knowing they are infected, getting ART, and getting PMTCT 101

Figure 7.2:   More testing, ART, and PMTCT reduce new infections and AIDS deaths 106

Figure 7.3:   Percentages of young women HIV-positive and maximum percentages of women HIV-positive by 5-year age cohort 112

Figure A1.1:   Percentages of women, men, and adults (aged 15 years and older) who are HIV-positive in the rest of the world, sub-Saharan Africa, South Africa, and Niger, 2019 119

Table A1.1:   Diversity of HIV/AIDS epidemics in sub-Saharan Africa, 2019 121

Figure A1.2:   Percentages of adults HIV-positive vs. percentages who mention sharing razors as a risk 122

Table A1.2:   Numbers of adults and children HIV-positive, AIDS-related deaths, and AIDS deaths as percentages of all deaths in sub-Saharan Africa, 1990-2019 125

Figure A1.3:   South Africa: Rapid epidemic onset, then life-saving treatments 126

Table A2.1:   Five studies that followed HIV-negative adults not aware their spouses were HIV-positive 133

Table A2.2:   Foreign organizations funding and approving the projects discussed in this annex..138

Acronyms

ANC	antenatal care
ART	antiretroviral treatment
CDC	Centers for Disease Control and Prevention
DRC	Democratic Republic of the Congo
ECHO	Evidence for Contraceptive Options and HIV Outcomes
EPI	Expanded Programme on Immunization
IDU	injection drug user or use
IV	intravenous
MSM	men who have sex with men
NET-EN	norethindrone enanthate
PMTCT	prevention of mother to child transmission
PP	post-partum
SIGN	Safe Injection Global Network
UN	United Nations
UNAIDS	Joint United Nations Programme on HIV/AIDS
UNFPA	United Nations Population Fund
UNICEF	United Nations Children's Fund
US	United States
WHO	World Health Organization

CHAPTER ONE

Purpose and outline

An HIV infection in a baby with an HIV-negative mother cannot be explained by mother-to-child transmission. An infection in a spouse whose only lifetime sex partner is HIV-negative cannot be explained by sexual transmission.

There are explanations, of course. Each such infection likely came from HIV-contaminated blood through some skin-piercing procedure – injection, infusion, tattooing, dental care, or other – with reused and unsterilized instruments. But until someone finds the source, the infection is unexplained. And whatever facility and procedure caused it may continue to infect others.

Purpose of this book

I hope the information here will help people who know about one or more unexplained HIV infections in their families and friends to mobilize community and government efforts to find and fix whatever caused the infections. The intended audience for this book includes teachers, reporters, clergy, local leaders, activists, lawyers and others in the general population. Although I have not written for health professionals, I expect many will be interested in the issues discussed here and may be ready to support investigations.

This book is for and about sub-Saharan Africa because that is where people have the biggest risk to get HIV from health care. Skin-piercing medical procedures are unreliably sterile in other countries as well, but because HIV infections are less common outside Africa, reused instruments are less likely to carry any HIV that could infect subsequent patients. Patients in Africa and elsewhere face other risks in health care, including hepatitis B and C infections from contaminated skin-piercing instruments, wrong diagnoses, and other errors, but that is too much to discuss in one book. I focus on unexplained HIV infections in sub-Saharan Africa.

Investigating unexplained infections

Outside sub-Saharan Africa

During 1986-2020, in dozens of communities across Asia, Europe, North Africa, the Americas and Australia, people who recognized unexplained HIV infections mobilized communities and governments to dig for answers, to find and fix the problem. In 12 cases, the resulting investigations uncovered large outbreaks, each with more than a hundred to as many as 100,000 HIV infections from medical procedures (see details in Chapter 2).

In some cases, as in Russia in 1988, government healthcare staff and officials were the first to recognize and respond. In other cases, investigations began informally in the community. For example, in the town of Ratodero, Pakistan, in 2019, a private doctor found one unexplained infection and arranged tests to find more. And in Roka, Cambodia, in 2014, a village leader with an unexplained HIV infection alerted others to go for tests. People who considered themselves at risk went for tests, finding more infections.

In Pakistan and Cambodia, increasing numbers of unexplained infections found through local informal investigations got the attention of the media and government officials, bringing government support for expanded investigations. In Libya in 1998, government got involved after parents appealed directly to Libya's leader, Muammar Gaddafi.

One unexplained infection may be the tip of an iceberg

Investigating a few unexplained infections may uncover many more. There are several reasons bloodborne HIV infections often come in bunches. Transmission may be going through multiple facilities. When doctors and nurses in one hospital or clinic are careless, similar attitudes and errors may be common in the region.

Whether one or more facilities are involved, transmission may be going through people who get multiple skin-piercing procedures. If someone gets HIV from a clinic or hospital and then goes for another treatment weeks later with a new (acute) infection, their blood would have a lot of HIV (high viral load). During the next treatment, their blood can get on instruments, and from those instruments get into and infect others. People getting repeat medical procedures include, for example, pregnant women, people with long-term health problems, inpatients, and persons selling blood or blood plasma.

How to get investigations started in sub-Saharan Africa?

Government officials in sub-Saharan Africa have recognized thousands of unexplained HIV infections over more than three decades without anyone ordering an investigation (Chapters 3-5). Hence, the Russian example, where government took the lead, may not apply to Africa. Other countries suggest a way forward. As in Pakistan, Cambodia, and Libya, the initiative for investigations in sub-Saharan Africa may come from communities. How might that happen?

Over the years, hundreds of thousands of people across sub-Saharan Africa have been aware of unexplained HIV infections in themselves, partners, children, and friends. Given the shame around HIV, and the fear of being accused of sexual misbehavior, many who have unexplained infections have swallowed their pain, not telling people they are infected or how they might have gotten HIV. This silence may not survive. More people are getting tested. This will not only expose more unexplained infections, but may also lead to wider awareness of how common HIV infections are in the general population, which may also challenge and diminish the silence and shame around HIV.

Community response depends not only on people recognizing and talking about unexplained infections, but also on people realizing that such infections are evidence they too are at risk. What will alert people to risks? When one or more young children are found with unexplained HIV infections, people may realize their own children are at risk. When one or more pregnant women or new mothers find they have unexplained infections, especially new infections, people might wonder about risks when they or other family members go for antenatal (pregnancy) care and delivery.

As more people become aware of unexplained infections and bloodborne risks, local informal leaders may emerge to guide the process of getting and sharing information, finding more unexplained infections, and developing ideas about where they are coming from and how to stop the source. Local leaders may be clergy, private doctors, HIV counselors, local officials, and others. As people continue to talk and test and to find more unexplained infections, sooner or later, local media can be expected to hear about and to report what is happening. One way or another, information about unexplained infections and community concerns will reach government officials. What happens next?

Communities aware they are at risk will then face whatever objections government officials might have to investigations. Health departments might not want to investigate, afraid they will find many more unexplained infections. Presidents and governors might not want to rock the boat by ordering health departments to investigate. Based on what has happened in other countries (Chapter 2), this is a challenge communities can win. With media attention, public pressure can build for governments to investigate to protect public health.

Based on experiences outside Africa, government decisions to investigate may come from outside the ministry of health – ministries of health taking orders from their government bosses (Chapter 2). In Kyrgyzstan, the president's office ordered the investigation. In Libya, Gaddafi ordered an investigation, over-ruling government's initial attempts to cover-up unexplained infections. In Romania, government's initial opposition to an ongoing informal investigation turned to support after a 1989 rebellion removed President Nicolae Ceausescu.

What happens during an investigation?

As communities and governments outside Africa have demonstrated time and again, investigations are not difficult in a technical sense. The basics are common sense. To find and fix mistakes, investigations:

- Identified places where people with unexplained HIV infections might have been exposed to contaminated blood.
- Tested others who had gotten skin-piercing procedures at suspected facilities.
- Found and corrected the procedures that were infecting people with HIV.

For what it's worth, the United Kingdom's Public Health England and the United States' (US) Centers for Disease Control and Prevention (CDC) advise how to investigate disease outbreaks from health care.[1,2] Their advice does not add much to what can be derived from using common sense and from reviewing what has been done elsewhere (Chapter 2).

Publicity is inevitable. When investigators invite patients treated at a hospital or clinic in recent months or years to come for HIV tests, such invitations get into the news. As the investigation proceeds, and as tests find and report more HIV infections traced to medical care, these unwelcome discoveries warn both patients and healthcare staff that something is wrong, and motivate changes to eliminate risks. In this way, publicity helps to get the best possible outcome.

To help people in affected communities resist shame and blame, health officials, media, HIV counselors, and others need to tell people clearly, insistently, and repeatedly that many if not most HIV infections in the community came from bloodborne risks, not sex. People also need to hear about how to recognize and avoid risks to get HIV from skin-piercing medical and cosmetic procedures.

In communities where several percent of the population has been infected for years, many of the unexplained infections uncovered in an initial informal investigation – and in any subsequent formal investigation – will be old infections from bloodborne risks years ago. Some new infections can be easy to spot, such as an HIV infection in a baby or young child with an HIV-negative mother, or in someone re-tested after an earlier HIV-negative test. But all unexplained infections, even those that may have been acquired years earlier (in spouses with no outside lovers, virgin young people, and older children) may point to facilities with unreliably sterile skin-piercing procedures and even ongoing risks.

In communities where many people are HIV-positive from old or new risks, one way to identify new infections is to sequence collected HIV samples (determine the order of each HIV's constituent parts). Because HIV sequences change over time as the virus multiplies in whoever it infects, most people with new infections from bloodborne risks will have HIV that is similar to HIV from several or many others infected from the same risks. Whoever is managing the investigation could arrange to have a laboratory sequence collected HIV samples. Sequencing is not expensive, and there should be no problem finding a laboratory to do it.

Investigations are decided and managed by communities and governments. Once things are underway, some governments have invited one or more international or foreign organizations such as the World Health Organization (WHO) or the US CDC to help. They have been followers, not leaders. Insofar as Africa is concerned, outbreak investigations may be more thorough and open if international and foreign organizations have less to say about how they are managed and reported. Because WHO, CDC, and other international and foreign health-oriented organizations have all along been aware that health care infects Africans (Chapter 3), they have a conflict of interest with respect to investigations. An investigation that finds a large outbreak will expose their long-term silence about the need for investigations to protect Africans.

How do investigations reduce bloodborne risks?

Outbreak investigations have revealed doctors and nurses being careless and cutting corners, for example, changing needles but reusing syringes for injections, or reusing plastic tubes or saline bags for infusions. Healthcare staff, even those not involved in an investigated outbreak, may realize that procedures they thought were safe enough may have infected patients. Investigations remind healthcare staff to practice what they have learned, to follow "standard precautions"[3] to protect patients.

Investigations may have their biggest impact for safety by alerting the public to pay attention to possible blood contact during skin-piercing events. People worried about safety may be afraid to go for vaccinations, antenatal care, and other procedures to protect their health. To allay fear, and to keep people coming to clinics and hospitals, providers will need to reassure patients they will be safe. An investigation thereby generates public pressure on healthcare managers and providers to respect patients' fears and to be more open with them. Providers may, for example, take new syringes and needles from sealed packages in front of patients, and take what is injected from single-dose vials (small bottles containing enough for one injection), so patients can rest assured that injections will not infect them.

People aware that reused skin-piercing instruments can transmit HIV can ask for sterile instruments in all settings, such as when getting an injection at a pharmacy, or when getting a manicure or tattoo. In this way, people aware of risks can enforce safe practices in settings beyond the reach of regulators, inspectors, and healthcare managers.

The changes needed to reduce bloodborne risks are not held back by budgets. Safer procedures may even save money, as when patients accept oral or no treatments instead of useless injections or infusions. What is needed is not more money but rather more transparency, accountability, and care to do things right (for example, sterilizing or at least boiling reused skin-piercing instruments).

Outbreak investigations demonstrate accountability in specific situations, but that is only a beginning. Getting healthcare providers and systems to be more accountable to patients is a process not an event. Do doctors, nurses, and health officials listen to patients and respect their concerns? Do they admit mistakes? Accountability is, by definition, a local challenge with local solutions. Foreign aid and advice are not needed and may get in the way. For decades, foreign aid agencies have pushed to extend specific healthcare interventions (vertical programs) even where agency staff are aware health care transmits HIV (Chapter 3). Donors' long-term support for one vertical program after another has undermined systems, safety, and accountability.

No fault investigations?

Keeping the focus on healthcare safety, the goal of investigations should be to find and fix errors, not to punish perpetrators or to compensate victims. Investigations that look for and find many or most people who have been infected in an outbreak can work backward from who was infected to pinpoint the facilities, procedures, and specific errors that allowed HIV to go from one patient or client to another. People found to be infected can be treated.

Speed saves lives. Finding all (or at least most) people who have been infected in an outbreak as fast as possible requires the cooperation of doctors and nurses, including those who infected patients through carelessness or ignorance but without any intent to harm. If such doctors and nurses are threatened with prison or financial ruin, they could be expected to obstruct investigations, thereby making it harder to find and treat victims and to find and fix mistakes.

Given the likely scale of HIV infection from health care over many years in sub-Saharan Africa, even multiple investigations could be expected to identify only a small fraction of healthcare staff who accidentally and carelessly infected patients. Prosecutions would, in practice, be arbitrary, going after whoever happens to be unlucky or powerless, especially low-income front-line staff, but missing managers and senior ministry officials who contributed to the problem by seeing and accepting risks and unexplained HIV infections for decades.

Similarly, given the likely scale of HIV transmission through unsafe health care over many years, even multiple investigations could be expected to find no more than a small fraction of victims. But even a small fraction would be too large for anyone – even government – to compensate except by offering free HIV care, which is already available to most if not all Africans with HIV from any risk.

In these circumstances, investigations could do a better job protecting public health if governments would legislate for no-fault investigations, with no liability for healthcare staff who cooperate. Since justice would not be achieved by selective prosecutions, no-fault investigations arguably promise the best justice available. No-fault investigations could be understood as a component of restorative justice,[4] helping healthcare workers recognize and admit what they have done, reducing harms from future health care, and finding and caring for victims.

Impact of investigations on Africa's epidemics?

For the purposes of this book, the contribution of unsafe health care to Africa's HIV epidemics does not have to be resolved. The point of the book is to encourage people who are aware of unexplained HIV infections in their communities to realize that whatever caused the infections threatens others, and to push for investigations to protect the community. Whatever might be the impact of an investigation on Africa's HIV epidemics is not their concern, and is not relevant to their asking for government to investigate.

What will be the impact of investigations on Africa's HIV epidemics? That is a secondary and controversial issue. The first issue is to protect the public's health. But for those interested, I consider the evidence in Chapters 6 and 7 and Annex 1.

Outline of this book

Preceding paragraphs describe what people can do to protect themselves, family members, and others in the community from getting HIV from health care and cosmetic services: When you see one or more unexplained infections, begin informal investigations in the community, and ask governments to help. Remaining chapters describe the challenges people may face when they ask for investigations and provide examples and information to overcome those challenges. The details of what happens next – what communities and governments do to stop HIV transmission through health care and to make healthcare staff and agencies more accountable to the public – will not and cannot be resolved before investigations begin and are, therefore, not discussed here.

Chapter 2: Investigations outside sub-Sahara Africa

During 1986-2020, governments outside sub-Saharan Africa investigated unexplained infections. Twelve investigations uncovered large outbreaks. For each of these 12 investigations, Chapter 2 reports who called attention to unexplained infections, how governments got involved, and what the investigations found.

Chapter 3: Bad advice for Africa: ignore HIV from health care

Beginning with some of the earliest research on HIV in Africa in the mid-1980s, international and foreign organizations and experts have advised Africans to accept and ignore unknown numbers of HIV infections from health care.

Chapter 4: No investigations in sub-Saharan Africa

No government in sub-Saharan Africa has investigated any unexplained infection by tracing and testing others who attended suspected source facilities. This failure is particularly striking in South Africa, with its terrible epidemic despite the country's economic and scientific resources.

Chapter 5: A large and ignored outbreak

Reported evidence suggests bloodborne risks caused a large HIV outbreak infecting hundreds of people in KwaZulu-Natal during 2013-14. The unexplained infections in this outbreak, and the inadequate responses by experts and the government, are outstanding examples of what has been going on for decades.

Chapter 6: How much HIV comes from sex?

For people who are aware of unexplained infections in themselves, family, and friends, the widely accepted myth that sex accounts for almost all HIV infections among adults in Africa has been an obstacle to getting others to believe unexplained infections are not from denied sexual risks. Chapter 6 provides evidence and references that people aware of unexplained infections can use to challenge that myth, to help others see that bloodborne risks infect a lot of people, and to recruit their support for investigations.

Chapter 7: Critical overview of responses to HIV in Africa

For almost 20 years, the international response to Africa's HIV/AIDS epidemics was a disaster. Beginning early in the twenty-first century, this began to change with belated promotion of testing and treatment. On the other hand, prevention has lagged. Donors and governments have continued to overlook HIV infections from health care. And they have proposed dangerous and unnecessary interventions for HIV-negative people – surgeries and drugs with side-effects – to protect them from getting HIV via sex.

Annexes

Annex 1 provides a thumbnail sketch of HIV epidemics in Africa. Topics include: differences between epidemics in sub-Saharan Africa vs. the rest of the world; epidemic diversity across Africa; and changes over the last three decades in the number of people living with HIV and numbers of AIDS deaths.

Annex 2 reviews unethical HIV research in Africa. Many of the foreign organizations and experts that have influenced the response to Africa's HIV epidemics have been neck-deep in unethical HIV-related research in Africa. Such research shows a double standard for Africa that parallels donors' double standard to see and accept HIV from health care in Africa but not in their own countries.

References

[1] Public Health England. *Communicable Disease Outbreak Management: Operational Guidance*. London: Public Health England, 2014.

[2] Centers for Disease Control and Prevention (CDC). Steps for investigating an infection control breach. CDC [internet], 27 February 2012. Available at: https://www.cdc.gov/hai/outbreaks/steps_for_eva l_ic_breach.html (accessed 31 July 2020).

[3] International Society for Infectious Diseases (ISID). *Guide to Infection Control in the Healthcare Setting*. ISID [internet], 2019. Available at: https://isid.org/guide/ (accessed 19 September 2020).

[4] Gabagambi JJ. A comparative analysis of restorative justice practices in Africa. Hauser Global Law School Programme [internet], October 2018.
Available at: https://www.nyulawglobal.org/globalex/Restorative_Just ice_Africa.html (accessed 3 September 2020).

CHAPTER TWO

Investigating Unexplained HIV Infections outside Sub-Saharan Africa

Soon after AIDS was first recognized in 1981, disease experts guessed it was caused by a virus. By 1985, scientists had found the virus and developed tests to see who was infected. Most people found to be HIV-positive with the new tests had expected risks (sex risks, injection drug use [IDU], or infected mothers). However, tests also found HIV-positive people without expected risks. Chapters 3-5 describe responses to unexplained HIV infections in sub-Saharan Africa. This chapter describes responses in the rest of the world.

During 1986-2020, governments outside sub-Saharan Africa investigated unexplained infections to find dozens of small to large outbreaks from unsafe medical procedures. For example, an unlicensed healthcare provider (quack) infected more than 50 people in an outbreak discovered in India in 2017[1]; and three clinics providing renal dialysis (to clean blood) infected about 80 patients in Egypt in an outbreak discovered in 1990.[2] (This website[3] gives details and references for these and many other outbreaks.)

Table 2.1: Investigated outbreaks with more than 100 HIV infections

Country, year the outbreak was discovered	Who was infected	Number of Cases
Pakistan, Ratodero, 2019	All ages, mostly children	1,250*
Pakistan, Kot Imrana, 2018	All ages, more women, children	~669
Cambodia, 2014	All ages	~240
Uzbekistan, 2008	Inpatient children	147
Kyrgyzstan,2007	Inpatient children	~270
Kazakhstan,2006	Inpatient children	118
Libya, 1998	Children	>120
China,1994	Plasma sellers	>100,000?
India,1989	Plasma sellers	~172
Romania,1989	Children	~10,000
Russia,1988	Inpatient children	>260
Mexico,1986	Plasma sellers	281

*This is from a January 2020 report (see text); the investigation was ongoing.
Sources: For each outbreak, see references in the text.

In 11 countries outside sub-Saharan Africa, investigations during 1986-2020 found 12 large outbreaks, each with more than 100 to tens of thousands of HIV infections from medical procedures (Table 2.1). This chapter focuses on these 12 outbreaks, with the following outline:

- Who recognized unexplained infections?
- When did government decide to investigate?
- What did the investigation find?
- What changed to reduce HIV from medical procedures?

The concluding section calls attention to some common issues relevant for sub-Saharan Africa.

Ratodero, Pakistan, 2019

Who recognized unexplained infections?

In early 2019, a private doctor in Ratodero, a town in Sindh province in southeast Pakistan, recognized an unexplained HIV infection:[4]

> It was a little girl... who first alerted him to the unseen outbreak. When she arrived at his clinic in late February [2019], she had a history of stubborn fevers that multiple doctors had been unable to relieve. Suspecting something was wrong with the 15-month-old's immune system, he sent her to a lab for an HIV test.

The test came back positive. The doctor had the parents and siblings tested. All were HIV-negative. "He began sending other patients for tests and was even more shocked by the results. In 20 days, 20 more patients had tested positive. He went to the town's local media." On 24 April 2019, local media broke the story.

When did government decide to investigate?

On 25 April, the day after television reports of unexplained infections in Ratodero, the Larkana district government and the district HIV/AIDS Control Programme arranged tests for parents of children found to be HIV-positive. When parents tested negative,[5] the Sindh Healthcare Commission and the HIV/AIDS Control Programme of Sindh province starting [*sic*] addressing the matter on a priority basis... [T]he entire vicinity was interviewed about their healthcare routine. They were also asked about the healthcare centres they visited in case of any ailment.

The Sindh Health Department launched "a mass screening program."[6] Government of Pakistan invited the US CDC, WHO, and other UN organizations to help with the investigation.[7]

What did the investigation find?

As of January 2020, more than 39,000 people had come for tests, of which 1,250 were found to be HIV-positive, including 985 children aged 0-15 years, 75 men, and 190 women.[8]

In June 2019, UNAIDS' regional director reported: "Unsafe injection practices including reuse of syringes and IV [intravenous] drips, both by the doctors as well as quacks [unlicensed healthcare providers] in addition to poor infection control have emerged as the leading causes of HIV outbreak in Ratodero..."[7] According to Fatima Mir, a member of the investigating team, "To call [infection control] abysmal doesn't even do justice to how bad it is... [T]here was a constant contamination of needles that were reused and reused and reused."[9]

Journalists helped to find and report what had happened. After the investigation began, a journalist who had helped to break the story realized that a doctor who had treated many children infected in the outbreak had treated his seven children as well. "He and his wife took them all to be screened and found his youngest daughter, two-year[s]-old... was positive."[4] Another parent with three HIV-positive children suspected their infections came from a doctor who had "applied the same drip on 50 children without changing the needle."[10]

Tests on 371 mothers of HIV-positive children found 39 were infected, of which six had HIV-positive husbands and eight had more than one HIV-positive child.[11] Because HIV infections were rare among pregnant women in the community (in 2011 only one in 2,990 had tested HIV-positive in the district's antenatal clinics[11]), the most likely way most if not all of these mothers got HIV is from breastfeeding their babies who got HIV from health care.[12]

What changed?[11]

> [T]he Sindh Health Care Commission... [closed] three blood banks... and almost 300 clinics run by untrained health-care providers... A special committee was established to address the inadequate infection control in health facilities and blood safety. As part of a community mobilisation campaign, formal meetings between community leaders, local government and health officials were held and HIV awareness sessions were done with community health workers including lady health workers, community-based organizations, law enforcement agencies, informal health-care providers (barbers), and registered health-care providers.

Kot Imrana, Pakistan, 2018

Who recognized unexplained infections?

In February 2018, a newspaper reported unusually large numbers of HIV infections in Kot Imrana village in Punjab province in eastern Pakistan. The issue had been discussed locally for some time. Reported numbers ranged from 37 to more than 250.[13]

When did government decide to investigate?

[E]lders of the area brought the matter [of large numbers of HIV infections] to the knowledge of Punjab government."[14] The Punjab AIDS Control Programme, responding to the elders' appeal, arranged tests for 2,717 residents of Kot Imrana; these tests found 35 to be infected.[14] Punjab provincial and Sarghoda district officials recognized the 35 infections as unusual, and no later than early March 2018 arranged expanded HIV testing in Kot Imrana.[15]

What did the investigation find?

By mid-March 2018, tests on 1,405 persons found 204 (14.5%) to be infected.[15] By January 2019, the District Health Department reported 669 (13.4%) of 5,000 residents of Kot Imrana were HIV-positive. HIV was more common in women and children. "[A] quack was found to have used the same syringe on multiple patients…" There were many quacks in the region. "[B]arbers are the other sources of HIV transmission because they use contaminated razors and blades."[16]

What changed?

I have found no account of what was done to improve infection control in the area.

Cambodia, 2014

Who recognized unexplained infections?[17]

> In late November, a 74-year old man from Roka commune [in central Cambodia], tested positive for HIV at the Roka Health Centre. After receiving his result, the man said he sent his grand daughter and son-in-law for testing and they also tested positive. Then the man stated he informed the other villagers that he had been receiving medical services from a private village practitioner and persuaded other villagers who had also been visiting the same practitioner to test for HIV.

When did government decide to investigate?

In early December 2014, local health authorities reported 30 unexplained HIV infections.[18] By 16 December, "An investigation team from MOH's [Ministry of Health's] National Centre for HIV/AIDS, Dermatology and STD... and University of Health Sciences" was in the district.[17] Within days, the provincial health department, the WHO, the US CDC, UNAIDS, the United Nations Children's Fund (UNICEF), and the Pasteur Institute in Cambodia joined the investigation.[17]

What did the investigation find?

Different sources report different numbers of HIV-positive persons found in the investigation. In mid-2016, Voice of America reported 292 infected.[19] The official investigation reports 242 HIV-positive persons identified through end-February 2015, of which 22% (52) were aged less than 14 years.[18,20] A comparison of HIV-positive residents with uninfected neighbors found that infected residents had received more injections, infusions, and blood tests.[21] Many persons with HIV were co-infected with the hepatitis C virus. Skin-piercing procedures are risks for both bloodborne infections. Unsafe health care had been spreading hepatitis C in the community for years before the HIV outbreak.[20]

Foreign organizations helping with the investigation sequenced several hundred HIV samples from the community (determined the order of HIV's constituent parts). Almost all sequences were very similar, showing fast transmission from one to 198 infections in an estimated 15 months from September 2013 to December 2014 (Figure 2b in[20]).

What changed?

Near the beginning of 2015, "the Health Ministry issued a directive to provincial health department officials, as well as provincial police and prosecutors, urging them to stop unlicensed health care workers from operating in their jurisdictions."[22] In 2017, "the MoH [Ministry of Health] is drafting new legislation to define and prohibit unlicensed practices."[21] Government sentenced one unlicensed healthcare provider (quack) in Roka to 25 years in prison and ordered him to pay compensation to 107 victims.[23]

Uzbekistan, 2008

Who recognized unexplained infections?

Hospitals in Namangan city and region in eastern Uzbekistan infected children as early as 2007.[24] One account says infections were discovered in October 2008,[25] but I have found no account of who recognized unexplained infections or when and how that happened.

When did government decide to investigate?

News from November 2008 reports an ongoing government investigation.[25] If the infections were discovered in October, then the investigation began almost immediately.

What did the investigation find?

The investigation found 147 children infected by contaminated instruments at multiple hospitals in the Namangan region in 2007-8. In 2009, the Uzbek government made a 21 minute film about the outbreak and subsequent investigation. The government then suppressed the film. However, someone passed the film to Ferghana News, which put it on the web in March 2010. According to the transcript, "medical workers... repeatedly reused medical instruments – catheters... and so on without sterilization and disinfection." One father recounts: "After the checks, it became clear that my son contracted AIDS due to the negligence of doctors who reused disposable syringes."[26]

Some mothers got HIV from their children (this report does not give a specific number[26]).

What changed?

The government sentenced 12 healthcare workers to 5-8 years in prison.[26] I have found no report of what was done to improve infection control.

Kyrgyzstan, 2007

Who recognized unexplained infections?

"Small numbers of children with nosocomial, or hospital-acquired, HIV infections began appearing in Osh Province [in southwest Kyrgyzstan] in 2004."[27] I have found no account of who tested the children and who determined that hospitals had infected them.

When did government decide to investigate?

Sometime before end-July 2007, a baby from Osh province tested HIV-positive at a hospital in Bishkek, the capital. This prompted the Ministry to send a commission to Osh to examine "all children who had been in contact" with the infected child in a hospital and clinic in Osh. Seven of 761 were found to be infected.[28] No later than 30 July, the president's office ordered prosecutors and the Ministry of Health to investigate.[29] Investigations expanded and continued at least into 2012.

What did the investigation find?

"The commission [that visited the two hospitals in July 2007] found that [disposable] subclavian catheters [tubes with needles to enter a vein] had been used many times."[30] By June 2009, the investigation had identified 72 HIV-positive children infected through health care.[31] In early 2012, the Kyrgyz Ministry of Health reported:[32]

> …it has so far tested 110,000 children in the area around the cities of Osh and Jalalabad and that it had found another 70 HIV positive children to add to the total of 200 cases already discovered. Several thousand more children need to be tested in the south of this rural, mountainous country.

In an incomplete account, 16 (22%) of 72 HIV-positive children had HIV-positive mothers,[31] likely from breastfeeding their infected children.

What changed?

In mid-2007, government dismissed several hospitals' chief doctors, the head of the regional blood transfusion center, and a sanitary official.[30] As of early 2012, the government had sentenced six health officials to three years in prison, and eight more were awaiting trial.[32] Aside from personnel changes and prosecutions, I have found no information about steps taken to improve infection control.

Kazakhstan, 2006

Who recognized unexplained infections?

During January-June 2006, 15 HIV-positive children were found in children's hospitals in Shymkent, a city in southern Kazakhstan.[33]

When did government decide to investigate?

Responding to unexpected infections, Kazakhstan's Health Protection Ministry sent a commission to Shymkent no later than mid-July 2006.[34]

What did the investigation find?

In June 2007, Kazakh officials reported the investigation had tested more than 10,000 children and had found 118 to be HIV-positive. The infected children had been treated at three children's hospitals.[35] Testing continued. In mid-2006, the Kazakh Health Minister said:[36]

> investigators may have found the cause of the infection and the reason why it spread. "In one of the children's hospitals there are 150 beds and only 13 catheter [tubes with needles to enter veins]... They are using these catheters without any disinfection.

Further investigation confirmed mistakes with catheters:[33]

> In hospitals, unsafe techniques for administration of IV [intravenous] medications and the use of reusable equipment for catheterization were observed... [A]dministration of IV fluids and SVC [catheters] were associated with infection among children, possibly because of unsafe practices.

Fourteen mothers of HIV-positive children were also HIV-positive. They most likely got infected while breastfeeding their children.[12,35]

What changed?

"After news of the first cases broke last year [2006], President Nursultan Nazarbaev ordered an overhaul of the health-care system and better checks on the quality of blood in the country's blood banks."[35] Seventeen healthcare workers were sentenced to nine months to eight years in prison.

Libya, 1998

Who recognized unexplained infections?

Staff of Al Fatah Children's Hospital in Benghazi, a coastal city in eastern Libya, identified HIV-positive children as early as mid-1998. I have not found an account of when or how parents learned their children were infected. In late 1998, La, a Libyan magazine, reported children with HIV infections suspected to have come from the hospital. The government closed the magazine.[37]

When did government decide to investigate?

"In November 1998 a group of desperate fathers interrupted a medical conference Gadhafi was attending in Benghazi and appealed to him for help."[37] Responding to the fathers, Gaddafi ordered an investigation.

What did the investigation find?

By early 1999, after testing "the majority of the children admitted to BCH [Benghazi Children's Hospital] during 1997 and 1998" the investigation had found more than 400 to be infected.[38]

At the request of the government, two foreign experts, Luc Montagnier and Vittorio Colizzi, assessed the evidence. Their 2003 report recognizes 404 children infected from health care. From a review of the children's medical records and other evidence, they concluded that HIV transmission began in the hospital in 1997 or earlier and may have continued into 1999.[39] Another study that looked at HIV samples from children infected in the outbreak estimated (from differences among the viruses, which change over time) that HIV transmission in the hospital began no later than 1997.[40]

At least 18 mothers of HIV-positive children were also infected. Most mothers likely got HIV by breastfeeding their children, who had gotten HIV from health care. Three mothers had received injections at Benghazi Children's Hospital.[41] The investigation found two nurses with HIV; one was likely infected through a needlestick accident and the other from health care at the hospital.[39]

What changed?

Transmission stopped soon after the outbreak was recognized, which points to better infection control. I have found no explanation of how that was achieved.

Gaddafi charged six foreigners (five Bulgarian nurses and a Palestinian doctor) working at the hospital with deliberately infecting the children, a charge that deflected attention from careless deficiencies in infection control. Mickey Grant reports much of this part of the story in *Injection!* a full-length movie.[42] Libya eventually deported the nurses and doctor.

China, 1995

Who recognized unexplained infections?

During 1990-94, companies and various government units established thousands of centers to collect blood plasma, often in poor rural areas.[43] Plasma (what remains after removing red and white blood cells) has various uses in medicine. Some of the collected plasma was intended for export.

"Officials first noticed a problem when batches of blood from… near Beijing, turned up carrying the AIDS virus at the end of 1994."[44] Also in 1994, a pharmaceutical company in Shanghai found that plasma bought from a woman in a nearby province was HIV-positive. Further testing in early 1995 confirmed she was infected along with two daughters who had also sold plasma; but her husband, who had not sold plasma, was HIV-negative.[45,46]

When did government decide to investigate?

Not later than early 1995, government officials recognized the contaminated blood discovered in late 1994 came from a large HIV outbreak caused by unsafe procedures to collect blood and plasma. I have found no account of how they came to that conclusion, but the timing is clear: In spring 1995 government closed all commercial plasma collection centers. Not later than 1997, government approved publicly reported research in affected counties.[43]

What did the investigation find?

I have not found any report of a comprehensive investigation. Journals and newspapers report pieces of the picture, such as results from testing people in one or more villages. For example, in a 1997 study in 18 villages, 75% of those who sold plasma at least ten times per month were HIV-positive.[43]

There is no clear picture of the number of blood and plasma sellers infected. China's Ministry of Health and UNAIDS estimated 55,000 former commercial plasma and blood donors were living with HIV in late 2005, and 10,000 former donors had died in 2005.[47,48] Many donors infected during 1990-95 would have died before 2005. If 55,000 is an accurate account of the number alive in late 2005, the number of blood and plasma sellers infected during 1990-95 likely exceeded 100,000.

What changed?

Government from early 1995 closed all commercial plasma collection centers.

India, 1989

Who recognized unexplained infections?

Not later than January 1989, doctors at the All-India Institute of Medical Sciences, a New Delhi hospital, found eight hemophiliacs to be HIV-positive. Weeks later, in early 1989, a doctor at the Institute had an Indian-produced blood product tested before giving it to his wife. It was HIV-positive. "Examination of more samples showed they were all positive for HIV."[49]

When did government decide to investigate?

In February 1989, government established a committee to assess HIV in blood products produced in India.[50]

What did the investigation find?

The committee found blood products from three of nine Indian companies were HIV-contaminated.[50] In July 1989, the National Institute of Virology reported 97 HIV-positive plasma donors in Pune, a city in western India, had been "most probably [infected] via a common source at any one of the commercial establishments where they sold their plasma."[51]

In early 1989, private doctors in Mumbai investigated another group of plasma sellers. Out of 200 tested, 86% (*circa* 172) were HIV-positive. Professional donors sold plasma an average of 3.5 times per week, and 90% had been doing so for five years.[52]

What changed?

In early 1989, government "ordered the withdrawal and destruction of all locally made blood products and banned their production until further notice."[50] To ensure safer blood products in the future:[49]

> [T]he health ministry has decided to step up its surveillance of blood products. It has also directed the Indian Council of Medical Research to investigate whether the procedures and technology used by the Indian manufacturers are adequate to ensure the safety of their products.

Romania, 1989

Who recognized unexplained infections?

In June 1989, doctors at Fundini Hospital in Bucharest tested some inpatient children for HIV.[53]

> Surprisingly, the first case tested, a 12-year old girl... was found to be seropositive. Subsequently, at that hospital 12 out of 30 children between 4 mo and 12 yr of age were found to be infected by HIV. Extending the study to other medical institutions, we [doctors] discovered more and more cases, suggesting an epidemic. Communication of these findings to the Ministry of Health resulted in the interdiction to cease conducting further studies. Despite warnings

from the Ministry of Health, we continued to test the infant population without reporting the results until December 1989, when the Communist regime in Romania collapsed.

When did government decide to investigate?

After the December 1989 revolt that toppled Ceausescu, government approved expanded testing.

What did the investigation find?

From June 1989 through May 1991, investigators tested 12,313 children aged 0-3 years, of which 1,382 (11.2%) were HIV-positive. Tests of 3,316 children aged 4-13 years found only 36 (1.1%) infected.[53] After much more testing, an estimated 10,000 children throughout Romania got HIV infections from health care during 1986-1992.[54] One possible explanation for the coincident onset of parallel outbreaks across Romania is that HIV somehow contaminated a Romanian-produced blood product (such as gamma globulin) that was distributed around the country.[55] According to this theory, some children got HIV from the infected blood product after which reuse of unsterilized instruments spread HIV from child-to-child, accounting for most infections.

In an incomplete account, 37 (7.5%) of 493 tested mothers of HIV-positive children were themselves HIV-positive. At the time, HIV was extremely rare in Romanian adults.[56] The most likely explanation for mothers' infections is child-to-mother transmission through breastfeeding.

What changed?

In 1989-90, Romanian and foreign non-government organizations began programs to improve infection control.[53]

The first and most efficient action was to inform the Romanian pediatric staff about pediatric HIV infection and that the source [*sic*] of HIV infection were blood and blood product transfusions, needles, and syringes commonly used repeatedly without being properly disinfected or sterilized, the treatment of malnourished children with whole blood [transfusions] to provide nutrients…, and multiple intramuscular injection instead of oral medication.

Russia (at the time, part of the Soviet Union), 1988

Who recognized unexplained infections?

Medical staff in Elista, a city in southwest Russia, found and reported two people with unexplained HIV infections: an inpatient child reported in November 1988 (both parents were HIV-negative); and a woman found HIV-positive about the same time through routine screening of blood donors (she had no HIV-positive sexual contacts).[57]

When did government decide to investigate?

Responding to reports of two unexplained infections, Moscow's Central Institute for Epidemiology began an immediate investigation, testing 12,000 people for HIV over the next two months.[58]

What did the investigation find?

From May 1988 through August 1989,[59]

> 288 Soviet citizens (265 children under 15 years of age and 23 adult women) were infected in 13 hospitals of Elista, Volgograd, Stavropol, Rostov-on-Don, Shakhty, Grozny, Astrakhan… All children and 1 woman were infected due to inadequate sterile technique, mainly by using shared syringes… Correlation of time of the patients' hospitalization to the foci and transfer of some of them to other hospitals pointed to one index patient of the outbreak – a child born to HIV-seropositive parents and admitted to Elista hospital in May 1988.

A Russian medical journal reports: "According to testimonies of mothers, medical personnel used the same syringes assigned for injections of the same medication, for example, gentamycin, for different children, replacing only needles…"[60]

Some babies infected their mothers: "22 women got most probably infected via breast-feeding their children having been infected in hospitals."[59]

Government extended testing throughout Russia: "Testing of 3,200,190 persons admitted to different hospitals in Russia in 1989 revealed other nosocomial foci [HIV transmission within hospitals]."[59] I have found no information about numbers and locations of infections not linked to Elista.

What changed?

"In all hospitals of the country strict control for rigorous aseptic technique, education of health-care workers and increase in number of disposable syringes were provided."[59]

Mexico, 1986[61]

Who recognized unexplained infections?

What was recognized initially was HIV-positive blood products. Beginning in May 1986, government ordered companies buying blood and blood plasma from donors to test the products for HIV and to report the results to the Secretariat of Health. By late 1986, government officials recognized a "steady increase" in HIV-contaminated blood products from a company buying plasma from people in a poor suburb of Mexico City.

When did government decide to investigate?

Acting on this information, in early 1987 the government began an investigation of the company's operations.

What did the investigation find?

A review of the company's records found 281 HIV-positive donors. Many infections were recent. Sixty-two donors had gotten infected during July-October 1986; the donor had an HIV-positive test after an earlier HIV-negative test. Investigators interviewed 54 HIV-positive and 58 HIV-negative donors. The biggest risk for infection was having donated often. Twenty percent of those donating 1-3 times per month were HIV-positive; 89% donating more than 10 times per month were HIV-positive.

What changed?

The government of Mexico banned commercial collection of blood and blood plasma.

Several take-aways from outbreak investigations

Investigations work!

In nine of the 12 outbreaks described in this chapter, multiple medical facilities infected patients and clients through carelessness. In Romania, for example, health facilities and orphanages throughout the country infected children during 1986-92. In Kyrgyzstan, an unspecified number of health facilities in the Osh region infected patients. In China during 1990-95, plasma collection centers in multiple provinces infected people selling plasma. Investigators traced infections to a single source in only three of the 12 outbreaks: one hospital (Libya), one company collecting blood plasma (Mexico), and one quack treating community residents (Cambodia).

Table 2.2: How many health facilities transmitted HIV, and what did the country's HIV epidemic look like in 2019?

Country, when the outbreak was discovered	Who transmitted HIV	% of adults HIV-positive in 2019
Pakistan, 2019	Many health facilities	0.1%
Pakistan, 2018	Many health facilities	0.1%
Cambodia, 2014	1 quack	0.5%
Uzbekistan, 2008	Multiple hospitals	0.2%
Kyrgyzstan, 2007	Multiple health facilities	0.2%
Kazakhstan, 2006	3 children's hospitals	0.3%
Libya, 1998	1 hospital	0.2%
China, 1994	100's of facilities collecting plasma	<0.1%
India, 1989	3 companies collecting plasma	0.2%
Romania, 1989	100's of health facilities, orphanages	0.1%
Russia, 1988	13 hospitals	1.2%
Mexico, 1986	1 company collecting plasma	0.2%

Sources: For each outbreak, see references in the text. Percentages of adults aged 15-49 years HIV-positive are from UNAIDS[62] except author's estimates for Russia, India, China, and Mexico.

Even where careless practices were widespread, the trajectories of HIV epidemics after investigations show little or no subsequent transmission through health care to the general population. In Romania, for example, only 0.1% of adults were HIV-positive in 2019, one of the lowest percentages in Europe. As of 2019, in nine of 11 countries with large investigated outbreaks, not more than 0.3% of adults were HIV-positive. In the other two, an estimated 0.5% were infected in Cambodia and 1.2% in Russia.

In 10 of the 11 countries, HIV circulates among IDUs and men who have sex with men (MSM), with little spread into the general population. Cambodia is the only one of the 11 countries where more women than men were HIV-positive in 2019 (according to UNAIDS estimates). Cambodia's 2014-15 investigation alerted people to risks to get HIV in health care, which has no doubt reduced those risks. If health care has gotten safer after 2014-15, this will likely change the sex ratio in coming years as fewer women and men get HIV from health care, while low numbers of men will continue to get HIV from IDU and MSM risks.

HIV transmits efficiently through skin-piercing procedures

In Cambodia, HIV went from one person to at least 198 within an estimated 15 months.[20] In Russia, HIV went from one child to 265 children within 16 months.[59] In these and other outbreaks, one patient infected one or more others, and they in turn infected others, and so on. For HIV to transmit to so many in such a short time, HIV from each infected person had to, on average, infect someone else within several months. In that time, how many skin-piercing procedures did an HIV-positive person get before reused instruments passed his or her HIV to someone else?

Over the years, WHO staff and consultants have given various estimates ranging from 0.3% to 1.2% for the risk to get HIV from a contaminated injection (0.5% in 1991[63]; 0.3% in 1999-2010[64-66]; 1.2% in 2004[67]; and 0.32%-0.64% in 2014[68]). With any of those estimates, the outbreaks discussed here were impossible. They would not have happened.

If, for example, the risk to transmit HIV through reused syringes and needles was 1.2%, then each HIV-positive person would have to get an average of 83 injections (83 x 1.2% ≈ 100%) for HIV to go through contaminated equipment to infect someone else. There was not nearly enough time. If it took 83 injections to transmit HIV from one person to another, transmission would take years, not weeks or months as in the investigated outbreaks.

The risk to transmit HIV through contaminated medical instruments had to be a lot greater than 0.3%-1.2% to generate these outbreaks. If, for example, the risk was 5%-10%, then reusing equipment after 10-20 procedures (20 x 5% = 100%; 10 x 10% = 100%) given to someone with HIV would on average transmit HIV to someone else. Are those numbers reasonable?

One of the opportunities for experts from WHO and elsewhere when they join an ongoing investigation is to collect information that could help to assess, find, and reduce bloodborne risks in other communities and countries. Some reports from these outbreaks list important risks, including IV [intravenous] drips and injections in Cambodia[21] and IV drips and catheters in Kazakhstan.[33] On the other hand, no one who helped with any investigation has used information from any outbreak to generate a realistic estimate of the risk to transmit HIV through injections or other medical procedures. In one report from Cambodia, experts from CDC, the Pasteur Institute, and WHO misleadingly downplayed bloodborne risks,[20] suggesting that HIV survives only a "few hours" in "needles/syringes." The study they cited to support that statement does not say that at all: the cited study[69] says HIV survives in syringes and needles stored at room temperature "up to 30 days, but generally 1-2 days."

In-country vs. foreign roles in outbreak investigations

People living in affected countries who were outraged about and/or afraid of HIV transmission through health care began all of the investigations described here. There is no indication any international or foreign organization helped to get things started by urging any government to investigate any unexplained infection.

When they have gotten involved, WHO, UNAIDS, CDC, and other foreign organizations have been followers, not leaders. One or more of these organization joined ongoing investigations in Kazakhstan, Kyrgyzstan, Cambodia, and Ratodero in Pakistan, but only after investigations were so far along they were going to expose large outbreaks.

Even after joining several ongoing investigations, no international or foreign organization has recommended similar investigations of unexplained infections anywhere else to protect patients. After the Cambodian outbreak, for example, experts from CDC, the Pasteur Institute, WHO, and elsewhere recommended efforts "to educate health care workers and communities at large on safe injection practices" but did not recommend outbreak investigations.[18]

Mismanaging an investigation

In early 2008, an HIV testing center serving Jalalpur Jattan town in northeastern Pakistan noticed an unusual number of people testing HIV-positive. To get more information, Pakistan's New Light AIDS Control Society, a non-government organization, worked with Punjab's Provincial AIDS Control Program to test 246 residents in June-July 2008; 88 tested HIV-positive. "One of the most important source [*sic*] appears to be... local medics (quacks) who have not been observing the sterilization and infection control techniques..." Two infected children had HIV-negative parents, and many women with no sex risks were infected.[70]

In response, Pakistan's Field Epidemiology and Laboratory Training Program (part of Pakistan's Ministry of Health, with support and advice from the US CDC) sent a team to Jalalpur Jattan to investigate. The team did not get to the town until five months after the 88 infections had been identified. Because it was fairly clear unsafe health care was the best explanation for many infections, the team should have asked infected people where they had received skin-piercing treatments and then invited others who had visited those places to come for tests. The team did not do that. It did not even contact the 88 HIV-positive people the New Light AIDS Control Society had identified.

Instead, beginning with a list of infected people provided by the local government hospital, the team tested relatives and looked for people with stigmatized behaviors (sex workers, MSMs, IDUs).[71] Overall, the team identified only 53 persons with HIV, including 26 previously tested. The team did not try to determine the extent of the outbreak and did not look for facilities providing unsafe skin-piercing procedures. This mismanaged investigation helped to keep people throughout Pakistan unaware of HIV infections from common blood-borne risks and was at least partly responsible for the subsequent large HIV outbreaks from medical care discovered in Kot Imrana in 2018 and Ratodero in 2019.

When babies are at risk, so are their mothers

Seven of the 12 large outbreaks reported in this chapter (in Russia, Romania, Libya, Kazakhstan, Kyrgyzstan, Uzbekistan, and Ratodero, Pakistan) infected mostly children. Information from all seven of these outbreaks report HIV infections in some mothers of HIV-positive children. Considering how rare HIV infections were in the general population in all seven countries, and especially in women, the most likely way most infected mothers got HIV was from breastfeeding their HIV-positive children. Child-to-mother transmission is efficient. A review of information from the Russian and Libyan outbreaks estimates that 40%-60% of children who breastfed after getting HIV infections from health care infected their mothers.[12]

References

[1] Unnao chief medical officer alerted in July about quack who caused HIV infections: Indian Express. *Scroll-in* [online], 11 February 2018. Available at: https://scroll.in/latest/868274/unnao-chief-medical-officer-alerted-in-july-about-quack-who-caused-hiv-infections-indian-express (accessed 12 October 2020).

[2] Hassan NF, El Ghorab NM, Rehim MSA, et al. HIV infection in renal dialysis patients in Egypt. *AIDS* 1994; 8: 853.

[3] Gisselquist D, Collery S. Unexpected HIV infections and HIV outbreaks from healthcare. *Bloodborne HIV* [internet] 2011-2020. Available at: https://bloodbornehiv.com/cases-unexpected-hiv-infections/ (accessed 12 October 2020).

[4] Farmer B. Cast out by HIV: how hundreds of children have been infected. *The Telegraph* [internet] 2020. Available at: https://www.telegraph.co.uk/news/pakistans-hiv-outbreak/ (accessed 12 October 2020).

[5] Siddique MN. HIV infections in Larkana. *Daily Times* 20 May 2019.

[6] Bhatti MW. 62 children tested HIV positive in Larkhana. *TheNews* 2 May 2019.

[7] Bhatti MW. UNAIDS delegation briefs Sindh Governor of causes of HIV outbreak in Ratodero, Larkana. *TheNews* 14 June 2019.

[8] Dawoodpoto J. 1,250 HIV cases reported in Ratodero in eight months. *Daily Times* 20 January 2020.

[9] Green A. HIV epidemic in children in Pakistan raises concern. *Lancet* 2019; 393: 2288.

[10] Gregory A. Nearly 900 children test positive for HIV in Pakistan after doctor "reuses syringes." *Independent* 27 October 2019.

[11] Mir F, Mahmood F, Siddiqui AR, et al. HIV infection predominantly affecting children in Sindh, Pakistan, 2019: a cross-sectional study of an outbreak. *Lancet Infect Dis* 2020; 20: 362-370.

[12] Little KM, Kilmarx PH, Taylor AW, et al. A review of evidence for transmission of HIV from children to breastfeeding women and implications for prevention. *Pediatr Infect Dis J* 2012; 31: 938-942.

[13] Niazzi SA. A Sargodha village under the shadow of HIV/AIDS. *Dawn* 20 February 2018.

[14] HIV, AIDS outbreak in Kot Momin village alarms residents, health officials. *Pakistan Observer* 1 March 2018.

[15] 204 patients test positive for HIV/AIDS in Sarghoda. *Dunya News* 19 March 2018.

[16] Wahid B. An update on the severe outbreak of HIV in Kot Imrana, Pakistan. *Lancet Infect Dis* 2019; 19: 241.

[17] Sarath E. HIV cases in Sangke district, Battambang. Ministry of Health, Cambodia [internet], 24 December 2014. Available at: http://www.cdcmoh.gov.kh/97-hiv-cases-in-sangke-district-battambang (accessed 12 October 2020).

[18] Vun MC, Galang RR, Fujita M, et al. Cluster of HIV infections attributed to unsafe injections practices – Cambodia December 1, 2014-February 28, 2015. *MMWR Mor Mortal Wkly Rep* 2016; 65: 142-145.

[19] Reaksmey H. Two years on, Roka villagers wait for justice, compensation. *VOA Khmer* [internet] 29 June 2016. Available at: https://www.voacambodia.com/ (accessed 12 October 2020).

[20] Rouet F, Nouhin J, Zheng D-P, et al. Massive iatrogenic outbreak of human immunodeficiency virus type 1 in rural Cambodia, 2014-2015. *Clin Infect Dis* 2018; 66: 1733-1741.

[21] Saphonn V, Fujita M, Samreth S, et al. Cluster of HIV infections associated with unsafe injection practices in a rural village in Cambodia. *J Acquir Immune Defic Syndr* 2017; 75: e82-e86.

22 Consiglio A, Pisey H. Government targets unlicensed medics amid HIV outbreak. *The Cambodia Daily* 5 January 2015.

23 Sovuthy K, HIV-positive widow dies in Roka commune. *Khmer Times* 10 January 2018.

24 Mirovalev M. Film: 147 toddlers infected in Uzbek HIV outbreak. *Seattle News 23* March 2010.

25 Vennard M. Uzbek children in "Aids outbreak." *BBC News* 11 November 2008.

26 The secret of Namangan-2008: two years since mass HIV inspection at children's hospital. *Fergana.News* [internet] 23 March 2010. Available at: http://enews.fergananews.com/article.php?id=2611 (accessed 24 September 2020).

27 Schenkkan N. Kyrgyzstan: HIV infections highlight systemic hospital breakdowns. *Eurasianet* [internet] 20 December 2011. Available at: https://eurasianet.org/kyrgyzstan-hiv-infections-highlight-systemic-hospital-breakdown (accessed 12 October 2020).

28 The Minister of Health told the details about infecting 11 people from the Nookatski Rayon with HIV/AIDS. *AKI Press* 31 July 2007.

29 Probe ordered in Kyrgyzstan HIV outbreak. *Radio Free Europe* 30 July 2007.

30 Re-using disposable equipment causes HIV outbreak in Kyrgyzstan. *RIA Novosti* 31 July 2007.

31 AP/Houston Chronicle examines HIV outbreak among 72 children, 16 mothers in Kyrgyzstan. *Kaiser Health News* [internet] 11 June 2009. Available at: https://khn.org/morning-breakout/dr00051491/ (accessed 12 October 2020).

32 Kilner J. Kyrgyz officials say another 70 children are infected with HIV/AIDS virus. *The Telegraph* 6 February 2012.

33 Sailybayeva GJ, Kaspirova A, Kuatbayeva A, et al. Human immunodeficiency virus (HIV) outbreak investigation among hospitalized children — Shymkent City, Southern Kazakhstan Region, June-November 2006. *57th annual EIS conference*, Atlanta, Georgia, 22-24 April 2009.

34 Pannier B. Kazakhstan: 14 children infected with HIV in hospitals. *Radio Free Europe* 21 July 2006.

35 Magauin E. Kazakh health workers jailed over HIV-infected children. *Radio Free Europe* 27 June 2007.

[36] Pannier B. Kazakhstan: HIV scandal sparks search for those responsible. *Radio Free Europe* 17 September 2006.

[37] Abu-Nasr D. AIDS scandal in Libya. *CBS News* 20 September 2001.

[38] Visco-Comandini U, Cappiello G, Liuzzi G, et al. Monophyletic HIV type 1 CRF02-AG in a nosocomial outbreak in Benghazi, Libya. *AIDS Res Hum Retroviruses* 2002; 18: 727-732.

[39] Montagnier L, Colizzi V. Final Report of Prof. Luc Montagnier and Prof. Vittorio Colizzi to Libyan Arab Jamahiriya on the Nosocomial HIV infection at the Al-Fateh Hospital, Benghazi, Libya (Paris, 7 April 2003). Webcite [internet], 14 February 2007. Available at: http://www.webcitation.org/5Mempgl11 (accessed 7 September 2020).

[40] de Oliveira D, Pybus OG, Rambaut A, et al. HIV-1 and HCV sequences from Libyan outbreak. *Nature* 2006; 444: 836-837.

[41] Visco-Comandini U, Longo B, Perinelli P. Possible child-to-mother transmission of HIV by breastfeeding. *JAMA* 2005; 294: 2301-2302.

[42] Grant M. *Injection!* Mickey Grant Films, 2006. Available at: https://www.youtube.com/watch?v=W00Kvn3T92g (accessed 20 July 2020).

[43] Wu Z, Rou K, Detels R. Prevalence of HIV infection among former commercial plasma donors in rural eastern China. *Health Pol Planning* 2001; 16: 41-46.

[44] Pomfret A. The high cost of selling blood: as AIDS crisis looms in China, official response is lax. *Washington Post* 11 January 2001.

[45] Wu Z, Liu Z, Detels R. HIV-1 infection in commercial plasma donors in China. *Lancet* 1995; 346: 61-62.

[46] Wu Z, Chen J. Scott SR, et al. History of the HIV epidemic in China. *Curr HIV/AIDS Rep* 2019; 16: 458-466.

[47] Lu F, Wang N, Wu Z, et al. Estimating the number of people at risk for and living with HIV in China in 2005: methods and results. *Sex Transm Infect* 2006; 82 (suppl 3): siii87-siii91.

[48] Ministry of Health, People's Republic of China, UNAIDS, WHO. *2005 Update on the HIV/AIDS Epidemic and Response in China.* Geneva: UNAIDS, 2006.

[49] Jayaraman KS. Further fears in India. *Nature* 1989; 337: 496.

[50] Jayaraman KS. All suspect in India. *Nature* 1989; 338: 611.

[51] Bannerjee K, Rodrigues J, Israel Z, et al. Outbreak of HIV seropositivity among commercial plasma donors in Pune, India. *Lancet* 1989; 2: 166.

[52] Bhimani GV, Gilada IS. HIV prevalence in people with no fixed abode: a study of blood donorship patterns and risk determinants. *VIII Int Conf AIDS*, Amsterdam, 19-24 July 1992. Abstract MoC 0093.

[53] Patrascu IV, Dumitrescu O. The epidemic of human immunodeficiency virus infection in Romanian children. *AIDS Res Hum Retroviruses* 1993; 9: 99-104.

[54] Buzducea D, Lazar F, Mardare EI. The situation of Romanian HIV-positive adolescents: results from the first national representative survey. *AIDS Care* 2010; 22: 562-59.

[55] Apetrei C, Loussert-Ajaka I, Collin G, et al. HIV type 1 subtype F sequences in Romanian children and adults. *AIDS Res Hum Retroviruses* 1997; 13: 363-365.

[56] Hersch BS, Popovici F, Apetrei RC, et al. Acquired immunodeficiency syndrome in Romania. *Lancet* 1991; 338: 645-649.

[57] Belitsky V. Children infect mothers in AIDS outbreak at a Soviet hospital. *Nature* 1989; 337: 493.

[58] Medvedev ZA. Evolution of AIDS policy in the Soviet Union. II. The AIDS epidemic and emergency measures. *BMJ* 1990; 300: 932-934.

[59] Pokrovsky VV. Localization of nosocomial outbreak of HIV-infection in southern Russia in 1988-1989. *VIII Int Conf AIDS*, Amsterdam, 19-24 July 1992. Abstract PoC 4138.

[60] Pokrovskii VV, Eramova II, Deulina MO, et al. Intra-hospital HIV outbreak in Elista. *Zh Microbiol Epidemiol Immunobiol* 1990; 4: 17-23.

[61] Avila C, Stetler HC, Sepulveda J, et al. The epidemiology of HIV transmission among paid plasma donors, Mexico City, Mexico. *AIDS* 1989; 3: 631-633.

[62] UNAIDS. HIV estimates with uncertainty bounds 1990-2019. Geneva: UNAIDS, 2020.

[63] Heymann DL, Edstrom K. Strategies for AIDS prevention and control in sub-Saharan Africa. *AIDS* 1991; 5 (suppl 1): S197- S208.

[64] Kane A, Lloyd M, Zaffran M, et al. Transmission of hepatitis B, hepatitis C and human immunodeficiency viruses through unsafe injections in the developing world: Model-based regional estimates. *Bull WHO* 1999; 77: 801-7.

[65] Schmid GP, Buve A, Mugyenyi P, et al. Transmission of HIV-infection in sub-Saharan Africa and effect of elimination of unsafe injections. *Lancet* 2004; 363: 482-488.

[66] Safe Injection Global Network. *WHO best practices for injections and related procedures toolkit.* Geneva: WHO, 2010.

[67] Hauri AM, Armstrong GL, Hutin YFJ. The global burden of disease attributable to contaminated injections given in health care settings. *Int J STD AIDS* 2004; 15: 7-16.

[68] Pepin J, Chakra CNA, Pepin E, et al. Evolution of the global burden of viral infections from unsafe medical injections, 2000-2010. *PLoS One* 2014; 9: e99677.

[69] Thompson SC, Boughton CR, Dore GJ. Bloodborne viruses and their survival in the environment: is public concern about community needlestick exposures justified? *Aus NZ J Pub Health* 2003; 27: 602-607.

[70] New Light AIDS Control Society, Canadian Pakistan HIV/AIDS Surveillance Project. Outbreak investigation: Mohalla JogiPura, Jalal Pur Jatan, Distt Gujrat, Punjab. Unpublished, 2008. Available at: https://dontgetstuck.files.wordpress.com/2012/01/new-lights-hiv-outbreak-investigation-gujrat-pakistan.pdf (accessed 3 June 2020).

[71] Ansare JA, Salman M, Safdar RM et al. HIV/AIDS outbreak investigation in Jalalpur Jattan (JPJ), Gujrat, Pakistan. *J Epidemiol Glob Health* 2013; 3: 261-268.

CHAPTER THREE

Health Experts Advise Africans:
Ignore HIV from Health Care

For more than 30 years, international and foreign organizations and experts have advised Africans to ignore an undetermined number of HIV infections from health care. The last section of this chapter considers and critiques reasons for giving such bad advice – what were people thinking?

1984-86: Not investigating unexplained infections in children

During June-August 1985, researchers at Mama Yemo Hospital in Kinshasa, Zaire (currently the Democratic Republic of the Congo [DRC]), used newly-developed HIV tests to test in-patient children aged 2-24 months and their mothers for HIV.[1] Sixteen (6.2%) of 258 children were HIV-positive with HIV-negative mothers. Five of the 16 had received a blood transfusion. "For children with HIV-negative mothers, medical injections appeared to be the most important risk... Injections are often administered in dispensaries which reuse needles and syringes yet may not adequately sterilize their injection equipment."

During 1984-86, researchers in Kigali, Rwanda, tested mothers of 76 HIV-positive children with AIDS aged 1-48 months. Fifteen (20%) of 76 mothers were HIV-negative.[2] Only 6 of the 15 children with HIV-negative mothers had received blood transfusions.

If such unexplained infections had been found in children in the US, Belgium or France (the countries that paid for the research), parents, media, politicians, and health officials would have demanded investigations. Governments of both DRC and Rwanda chose not to investigate, which was their mistake. But that does not excuse the failure of foreign funders and researchers to recommend investigations to protect public health.

The research team in DRC recommended unspecified "public health measures" to prevent HIV transmission through injections and blood transfusions.[1] Researchers in Kigali recommended boiling or bleach to de-contaminate reused syringes.[3] But without investigations, such recommendations were unguided – there was no way to zero in on the errors that infected patients – and the public remained ignorant about what was happening and about bloodborne risks.

Only months after researchers reported unexplained infections in children in Mama Yemo Hospital in DRC, four of the same experts published an influential overview of AIDS in Africa. They expected bloodborne risks to continue: "one cannot hope to prevent reuse of disposable injection equipment when many hospital budgets are insufficient for the purchase of antibiotics."[4] Two authors of that overview led the international response to HIV/AIDS for 17 of the next 22 years: Jonathan Mann led WHO's HIV/AIDS programs during 1986-90; and Peter Piot led UNAIDS during 1996-2008.

In 1988, experts who had reported unexplained infections in children in Kigali published an overview of healthcare risks for HIV in Africa.[3] They expected continuing unknown numbers of HIV infections from health care: "The importance of medical injections in the epidemic of HIV infection seems to differ from one area to another." But they did not want people to be afraid: "The risk of HIV contamination is low, if any, and should not compromise the immense benefit that widespread immunization campaigns have on children's health."

1991-93: Safe for African children, not for UN employees

After investigations in Russia and Romania in 1988-90 found health care had infected hundreds to more than a thousand children with HIV (Chapter 2), WHO in 1991 arranged for hospitals in four countries in Africa – Rwanda, Tanzania, Uganda, and Zambia – to test inpatient children aged 6-59 months and their mothers for HIV. WHO reported combined data from the four countries. Sixty-one (1.1%) of 5,593 children were HIV-positive with HIV-negative mothers. Only three of the 61 had been transfused. At least four more children got HIV within three months after leaving the hospital. When reporting these 65 unexplained infections, WHO's Global Programme on AIDS assured: "Based on these studies, the risk of... patient-to-patient transmission of HIV among children in health care settings is low."[5] That statement says more about WHO's double standard for Africa than about risks to get HIV from health care in Africa.

About the same time that WHO's Global Programme on AIDS was assuring Africans they did not need to worry about getting HIV from health care, WHO was giving a different message to United Nations (UN) employees. WHO's 1991 booklet, *AIDS and HIV Infection: Information for United Nations Employees and Their Families*, advised employees[6]

> ...living or traveling in areas where the level of medical care is uncertain [to]... take special precautions to avoid HIV transmission via blood... The WHO medical kit contains... syringes and needles in case staff need to have blood taken or receive an injection or vaccination while traveling... If you are not carrying your own needles and syringes, avoid having injections unless they are absolutely necessary... Avoid tattooing and ear-piercing. Avoid any procedures that pierce the skin, such as acupuncture and dental work, unless they are genuinely necessary.

1987-99: Immunization programs deflect HIV worries

In 1974, WHO and partners established the Expanded Programme on Immunization (EPI). For more than a decade, immunizations lagged in Africa. A 1987 meeting of EPI's Global Advisory Group appreciated that 33% of children in Africa had received their third diphtheria, whooping cough, and tetanus (DPT) vaccination by 1986. The same meeting heard that only 42% of more than 400 immunization centers visited by WHO consultants in 39 African countries sterilized syringes between immunizations.[7] Despite such recognized risks, the meeting recommended: "Continued acceleration" of EPI programs "to meet the goal of Universal Childhood Immunization by 1990."

In a 1987 joint statement on immunizations, WHO and the United Nations Children's Fund (UNICEF) imagined a choice between unsafe injections and no immunizations. They opted for unsafe injections: "Halting immunization efforts because of the fear of AIDS would increase deaths among children, while doing little to stop HIV transmission."[8] That imagined trade-off ignored a third option: safe injections.

In 1989, foreign-funded health experts in Uganda worried that HIV prevention messages warning about risks to get HIV from injections would dissuade mothers from having their children immunized.[9] Based on that concern, a 1989 survey asked mothers if they thought injections could transmit HIV. Mothers aware of the risk were more likely to have had their children immunized. Despite that finding, and even though experts could not "rule out the occasional transmission of HIV via injections... radio messages about AIDS in Uganda have been modified to ensure that parents are aware of the safety of immunizations."

In 1994, WHO estimated that as many as a third of immunization injections were unsterile in four of WHO's six regions.[10] In the same year, the head of research at WHO's Global Programme on AIDS and the future head of UNAIDS worried that outbreak investigations, as in southern Russia in 1988-89, would alert people to bloodborne risks and thereby harm immunization programs:[11]

> The media, which has publicized HIV nosocomial outbreaks [i.e., outbreaks from hospitals], has helped to increase public awareness about the dangers of nosocomial transmission. But the short-term benefits of increased public awareness may not always be positive [*sic*]. The current outbreak of diphtheria in Russia... has been blamed in part on publicity surrounding nosocomial HIV transmission in southern Russia and other problems in the health-care system, which are thought to have discouraged mothers of young children from seeking immunizations from a health-care system that they perceived to be unsafe.

Already in July 1987, WHO staff had been reviewing various designs for syringes and needles that could not be reused, including "auto-destruct" syringes that would break or seize up after use, and pre-filled syringes.[12] But for various reasons, almost nothing happened until the end of the 1990s. As late as 1996, annual sales of auto-destruct syringes had reached only 60 million, equivalent to 6% of the estimated one billion immunization injections given annually in developing countries.[10] For more than a decade, public health officials did not adopt available and simple changes into immunization programs to protect children from unsafe injections.

1999-2003: Breakthrough discussions of HIV from health care

During 1989-98, seven surveys in African countries coordinated by WHO found that 20% to more than 90% of injections were unsafe. At the time, WHO kept most of those findings secret. But the evidence finally broke through. In 1999, the *Bulletin of the World Health Organization* published survey findings (but without naming many of the countries) along with another paper that used those findings to estimate unsafe injections caused 51,000-102,000 HIV infections in Africa in an unspecified recent year.[13,14]

In response to such worrisome information and estimates, WHO, UNICEF, and the United Nations Population Fund (UNFPA) issued a joint statement promoting auto-disable syringes for immunizations. That statement had teeth in the form of time-bound commitments:[15] "UNICEF announces that, as of 1 January 2001, no procurement service contracts for standard disposable syringes will be entered into... WHO, UNICEF and UNFPA urge that, by the end of 2003, all countries should use only auto-disable syringes for immunization."

However, immunizations accounted for only about 10% of all injections.[13] Most injections were curative; some delivered birth control. Thus, shifting immunizations to auto-disable syringes averted only a small part of the estimated health damage from unsafe injections.

Safe Injection Global Network (SIGN)

In 1999, WHO and CDC established the Safe Injection Global Network (SIGN) with a small staff and office in WHO. SIGN's agenda was to coordinate efforts to reduce all unsafe medical injections for all purposes.

Whereas donors funding immunization programs had leverage to promote auto-disable syringes for immunization, donors did not have similar leverage for other medical injections. However, the proposed solution was much the same. SIGN with WHO and donors urged governments and private providers to use auto-disable syringes or new disposable syringes and to sterilize any reused syringes and needles. In addition, SIGN and partners promoted programs to educate the general public to ask for fewer injections and to watch providers take new syringes and needles from sealed packages.

To improve injection safety over time, SIGN developed survey forms to collect information on injection practices, published survey findings, and arranged country-level and international meetings to discuss injection risks and remedies. Reviewing available information, SIGN estimated Africans in 2000 received an average of 2.0-2.2 injections per person per year, of which 17%-19% reused syringes and/or needles – more than 200 million injections per year with reused equipment.[16] From this, SIGN estimated unsafe injections caused 52,000-104,000 HIV infections (best estimate: 83,000) in Africa in 2000.[17]

WHO hosts a debate

During 2002-3, several medical journals published letters and articles calling attention to unexplained infections[18] and estimating – from evidence previously reported in medical journals – that unsafe health care and other bloodborne risks accounted for well over half of HIV infections in Africa.[19,20] In response, WHO hosted a closed-door meeting in March 2003 to discuss the evidence. The 20 attendees – WHO and UNAIDS staff and invited experts – discussed the percentages of HIV infections coming from injections and other bloodborne risks, with a focus on Africa. WHO's report from the meeting says attendees continued to disagree about how much medical injections contribute to Africa's HIV epidemics, but notes agreement on two points:[21]

> First, that better data on the possible role of unsafe injections, and other health care practices, in HIV transmission are needed... Second, that unnecessary injections should not occur and, whether in the formal or informal health sector, such injections should be safe.

US Senate hearings

Soon after US Senator Jeff Sessions heard about WHO's 2003 meeting on HIV infections from health care, he arranged two hearings in the US Senate to discuss HIV transmission through health care in Africa. With his leadership, the US committed $300 million over 2003-9 to improve the safety of medical injections and blood transfusions in 15 countries (12 in Africa, Guyana, Haiti, and Vietnam). The US allocated this money through programs managed by USAID, CDC, and other agencies.

2004: WHO and UNAIDS reaffirm their double standard for Africa

If there was any question about how well international acceptance of bloodborne risks and HIV transmission during health care in Africa survived discussions during 1999-2003, two publications in 2004 made it crystal clear the double standard survived. WHO and UNAIDS staff continued to accept that Africans were at risk to get HIV from health care, but they did not want UN staff to take the same risks.

In a prominent 2004 article in *The Lancet* medical journal, WHO and UNAIDS staff led a team of 15 authors assessing risks for Africans to get HIV from unsafe injections. None of the authors had expertise or responsibility for hospital infection control. Authors repeated WHO's estimate that Africans received more than 200 million injections per year with reused and unsterilized equipment, but assured: "Washing or, possibly, rinsing or soaking of syringes or needles will dilute any blood that might have contaminated the equipment."[22]

To their credit, the authors mentioned HIV outbreaks from health care in Russia, Romania, and Libya. But instead of acknowledging that those outbreaks came to light because governments investigated unexplained infections, and that African governments had not done so, they simply denied that what had happened there was relevant for Africa: "To believe [the risks demonstrated in those outbreaks] can be generalized to the African setting is... erroneous." The authors worried that US Senate "hearings to establish whether HIV/AIDS funds should be devoted to programmes that target unsafe injections" might interfere with efforts to reduce sexual transmission of HIV in Africa.

As noted above, in 1991 WHO published a booklet for UN employees, warning them to avoid skin-piercing health care in Africa. UNAIDS's 2004 revision of the booklet continued such warnings, but assured safe health care for UN staff:[23]

> In several regions, unsafe blood collection and transfusion practices and the use of contaminated syringes account for a notable share of new infections. Because we are UN employees, we and our families are able to receive medical services in safe health-care settings, where only sterile syringes and medical equipment are used, eliminating any risk to you of HIV transmission as a result of health care.

Why did the double standard survive?

During 1999-2003, experts in international meetings and medical journals bandied about estimates of more-or-less 100,000 Africans infected each year from medical injections. In many experts' home countries, such estimates would have brought outrage and immediate investigations to find and treat people who had been infected and to find and fix whatever had infected them. Experts talking about 100,000 infections per year from injections in Africa expected and ignited no such response.

Estimates of infections from injections in Africa were based, in part, on evidence-based estimates that 17%-50% of injections were unsafe.[14,17] In many experts' home countries, even if an unsafe injection does not infect anyone, it is considered a "near-miss," "close-call" or "potential adverse event" that should be investigated to find out why it happened and to prevent future mistakes.[24] A similar response was not considered for recognized unsafe injections in Africa.

In other words, much of the 1999-2003 discussion of HIV infections from health care in Africa was carried on within the framework of the double standard. Safe enough for you, but not for us.

Great progress with injections, but missing the big picture

Building on more than a decade of back-room debates about risks with immunizations injections, international health officials and experts who were most concerned about HIV from health care focused on injections. Long-term concerns about HIV and other bloodborne infections from unsafe medical injections broke through to public discussion and attention in 1999.

Attention brought change. The estimated annual number of unsafe injections per person in sub-Saharan Africa fell almost 90% from 2000 to 2011-15.[25,26] Some of this reduction was due to fewer injections, but most was due to less reuse. Although data for 2011-15 are weak (based on patients' recall for injections received months earlier), there has no doubt been a big drop in numbers of unsafe injections as well as in numbers of HIV (and hepatitis B and C) infections from injections.

But despite fewer unsafe injections, numbers of unexplained HIV infections have remained high (Chapters 4-6). Clearly, the focus on injections has missed the big picture. The decision to ignore medical procedures other than injections and transfusions was reached with insufficient evidence and almost no discussion. The variety and numbers of skin-piercing medical procedures that Africans receive have increased over the years. There is not even good information on what and how many procedures an average person receives in a year, much less on how often instruments are reused without sterilization. The best and quickest way to find such risks is to investigate unexplained infections – to trace infections to facilities and procedures. Outbreak investigations might also find risks with cosmetic procedures, such as tattooing, piercing, and manicures.

Getting providers to shift to auto-disable syringes was a supply-side, technical solution working through healthcare professionals. Some programs advised the public to watch providers take new syringes and needles from sealed packages and to take fewer injections. However, the emphasis was on supply-side interventions, leaving in place weak accountability to patients, which has been the core of the problem.

Even for injections, interventions were insufficient. For example, a parent taking a child for an injection might see the nurse take a new syringe and needle from a sealed package, but if the nurse then takes medicine to inject from an already opened multi-dose vial (with medicine for multiple injections), whatever is injected may have been contaminated by a previous syringe or needle withdrawing medicine from the vial. The risk that injections might transmit HIV could have been eliminated by shifting to either single-dose vials along with new (auto-disable) syringes or to pre-filled syringes.

Moreover, telling healthcare workers again and again how to give safe injections does not always work. Some people are careless, cutting corners and thinking what they do is safe enough. As of 2011-15, according to estimates reported above, Africans were still getting almost four million injections per year with reused syringes and needles.[26]

Critics missed the main point

During 1999-2003, I participated in discussions about HIV from unsafe health care in Africa. I did some short-term work for SIGN, co-authored papers in medical journals, presented at WHO's March 2003 meeting, and testified in the US Senate.

With hindsight, I am chagrinned we missed the main issue. We spent too much time debating the percentage of HIV infections coming from injections and other medical procedures. That percentage is important, but it is a secondary issue. When someone sees an unexplained HIV infection, the public health response – investigating to find and treat others infected from the same source and to find and fix the source – should be the same whatever the percentage of infections in the country or community coming from bloodborne risks.

Moreover, the failure to investigate unexplained infections was an objective failure. Debates about the percentages of HIV infections in Africa coming from bloodborne risks were a messy distraction that resisted resolution since many experts were willing to rely on weak evidence and jerry-rigged models (see Chapter 6). It was frustrating to tilt against wobbly arguments. But that was a sideshow. If the goal was to stop HIV transmission through health care in Africa, we did not need to win debates about estimated percentages. What we needed to do was to call attention to a simple fact: the failure to investigate unexplained infections.

If some of us involved in 1999-2003 discussions had prioritized investigations of unexplained infections, the immediate outcome might have been the same. Based on what has happened before and since, it seems likely that few of those involved in the discussions would have endorsed investigations. But persistently proposing and emphasizing investigations would have called attention to unexplained infections and challenged discussants to recognize investigations as an option. Such a discussion might have promoted parallel debates in communities and governments across Africa about whether to investigate unexplained infections.

International and foreign organizations are not the ones to manage investigations. That is for communities and governments. But what can such organizations and their associated experts say and do to encourage governments to investigate? And what should donors providing health aid do in countries where health care is a risk to transmit HIV? These issues are still pending.

2004-20: More evidence

Decisions made at the end of the 1980s and reconfirmed in 2004 – to accept undetermined numbers of HIV infections from health care in Africa – have stayed in place since. The double standard continues despite multiple large outbreak investigations in Asia (Chapter 2) and new evidence of healthcare risks and unexplained HIV infections in sub-Saharan Africa.

Not sterilizing reused instruments

After international organizations ramped up attention to unsafe injections in 1999-2003, nine African governments surveyed random samples of health facilities. Among other issues, surveys assessed facilities' ability to process instruments for reuse (with heat sterilization or high level chemical disinfection). Across the nine countries, 83%-98% of hospitals had equipment to process instruments for reuse (Figure 3.1). However, considering all healthcare facilities, including hospitals, clinics, and others, only 17%-94% had equipment to do so. But just having equipment did not ensure reused instruments were sterile. In some facilities, the worker responsible for operating the equipment was not aware of the correct processing time or temperature, and manuals were not available (Figure 3.1 ignores those deficiencies).

Figure 3.1: Percentages of health facilities with equipment to process instruments for reuse*

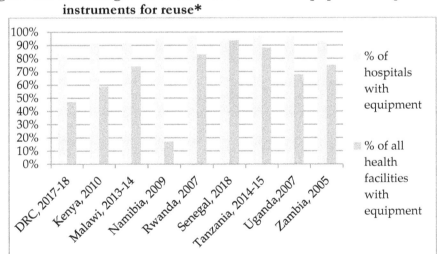

Abbreviations: DRC: Democratic Republic of the Congo. *Data from surveys after 2004, taking only the latest survey for each country.
Sources: DRC[27]; Kenya[28]; Malawi[29]; Namibia[30]; Rwand[31]; Senegal[32]; Tanzania[33]; Uganda[34]; Zambia.[35]

More unexplained HIV infections in Africa

Beginning in 2001, many countries in sub-Saharan Africa managed national surveys to test people for HIV. Surveys found and reported unexplained HIV infections in youth and adults who said they were virgins. Some surveys reported HIV in children with HIV-negative mothers. Because unexplained infections challenge African governments to investigate, I report such data in Chapter 4.

2004-20: More inadequate responses

World Alliance for Patient Safety

Responding to increasing concerns about healthcare providers not washing their hands, giving the wrong drugs, and other mistakes, WHO in 2004 established the World Alliance for Patient Safety. Among its other suggestions, the Alliance recommended reporting and learning from adverse events, such as unexplained infections:[36]

> A major element of programmes to improve patient safety is having the capacity and capability to capture comprehensive information on adverse events, errors and near-misses so that it can be used as a source of learning and as the basis for preventive action in the future.

The Alliance urged health facilities and ministries to investigate adverse events to find and fix mistakes.[24] The focus on adverse events was on target – a breath of fresh air!

However, the Alliance has ignored unexplained HIV infections in sub-Saharan Africa as adverse events. During its lifetime, the Alliance has been silent about investigations of large HIV outbreaks in Kazakhstan, Kyrgyzstan, Uzbekistan, Cambodia, and Pakistan. These tragedies are relevant for Africa. Experiences in these countries could provide guidance about how to work with the public during an investigation, how to improve healthcare systems, and how to continue high-priority healthcare programs. Neither the Alliance nor any of the foreign organization helping with recent investigations in Asia has proposed similar investigations in Africa.

Continuing a limited focus on injections

In 2015, WHO recommended countries to shift to "safety-engineered syringes" for most injections, not only immunizations.[37,38] Safety-engineered syringes are auto-disable syringes with additional features to protect healthcare workers from "needlestick accidents" (getting stuck with a used needle). Common designs to prevent needlestick accidents have a flap or sleeve to cover a needle after use. WHO's 2015 injection safety strategy parallels the strategy SIGN and partners promoted from 1999 for immunization injections: a technical solution that works through health professionals. The strategy ignores skin-piercing procedures other than injections and says nothing about investigating unexplained infections.

HIV prevention programs say little about HIV from healthcare

WHO's *Global Health Sector Strategy on HIV 2016-21* acknowledges (page 33[39]): "Although reliable data are lacking, it is likely that unsafe medical injections and blood transfusions account for significant numbers of new HIV infections." The strategy endorses WHO's 2015 injection safety policy (see previous paragraph). But HIV from health care is clearly not a big issue: the 50-page document commits only one paragraph and several clauses to healthcare risks. UNAIDS was even less attentive. UNAIDS' strategy for 2016-21 does not mention HIV from unsafe health care, medical injections, or transfusions.[40]

Scientific and medical elites avoid the obvious

Over the years, respected and influential organizations with deep involvement in Africa have been silent about unexplained infections. For example, in 1996, Harvard University with the government of Botswana established the Botswana-Harvard AIDS Institute Partnership, aiming "to develop interventions appropriate to stemming the epidemic."[41] Botswana has one of the world's worst HIV epidemics, with an estimated 20.7%-26.1% of adults HIV-positive during 1996-2019. As far as I have been able to see, for more than two decades, no one associated with Harvard's work in Botswana has asked about or said anything about bloodborne risks or unexplained HIV infections.

Partners in Health, a US-based non-government organization, has made major contributions to HIV treatment for Africans (see Chapter 7). At the request of the government of Lesotho, Partners in Health began working in Lesotho in 2006. According to UNAIDS estimates, 22.8%-24.6% of adults in Lesotho have been HIV-positive from 2006 through 2019.[42] During 14 years, Partners in Health staff have no doubt met and heard of many people with unexplained infections. But as far as I can see, no one associated with Partners in Health has mentioned such infections or asked for any investigation to find their source.

Much of what Harvard University and Partners in Health have done in Botswana and Lesotho is great, for example, helping to extend antiretroviral treatment. But by staying silent about unexplained infections and not urging investigations (at least not publicly), they have not protected people.

Why such bad advice?

Accepting that health care transmits HIV to an unknown number of people without asking for investigations or warning people at risk is inconsistent with health professionals' responsibilities as described in the World Medical Association's Declaration of Lisbon on the Rights of the Patient: "Physicians and other persons or bodies involved in the provision of health care have a joint responsibility to recognize and uphold these rights," including (article 1) "The right to medical care of good quality" and (article 9) "the right to health education that will assist him/her in making informed choices about personal health and about the available health services."[43] Not warning people about risks is similarly inconsistent with the Preamble to the Constitution of the World Health Organization: "Informed opinion and active co-operation on the part of the public are of the utmost importance in the improvement of the health of the people."[44]

Excuse for abuse

The priority for foreign health aid in sub-Saharan Africa has been to extend interventions – more children immunized, more pregnant women attending antenatal care, more hospital deliveries, more primary health care. A common excuse for discouraging outbreak investigations and for not telling people about risks to get HIV from medical procedures has been that warning people might scare them away from health care. This excuse:

- Does not respect the public's role in making health care safe. Not telling the public about risks in health care does not give them the information they need to help reduce those risks.
- Does not allow people to make their own choices. People should be informed and thereby allowed to decide for themselves if they would rather risk getting HIV from a specific healthcare procedure or risk the consequences from forgoing it.
- Assumes healthcare managers and patients have two choices: unsafe health care or no health care. This overlooks safe care as a third option.

For healthcare professionals, the excuse that warning people about risks might scare them away from health care is self-serving. Not warning protects medical professionals from accountability to patients, which might be uncomfortable. Other reasons for silence may be to protect their jobs or institutions by not saying something employers, funders, or supervisors might not want to hear.

Racial stereotypes and the white-savior complex

Most experts knowledgeable about HIV in Africa have by now accepted survey-based evidence that sexual behavior in Africa is not horrendously promiscuous. But among the European and American public, across the political spectrum from left to right, racial stereotypes of sexual behavior are still widespread. With such beliefs, the European and American public accepts that sex explains Africa's HIV epidemics. Such blindness among the public in donor countries protects the bad advice that international and foreign organizations have been giving Africans: ignore unexplained infections, accept unknown numbers of infections from health care, and focus on sexual risks.

Another problematic belief among Europeans and Americans is the white savior complex – that foreign aid can solve Africa's problems. Finding and stopping HIV transmission through health care does not need foreign aid. The solution requires healthcare managers and providers to be accountable to patients. Foreign aid can undermine that solution by strengthening accountability to paymasters, which can weaken accountability to patients.

Dissent

Not all health experts outside sub-Saharan Africa have gone along with the double standard. For example, 15 authors of two papers, in 2003[45] and 2009,[46] asked for outbreak investigations in Africa. Authors include the head of the International Clinical Epidemiology Network, editor of a medical journal, a staff of Physicians for Human Rights, professors at universities in India, Germany, and Ireland, members of other organizations, and independent experts.

References

[1] Mann JM, Francis H, Davachi F, et al. Risk factors for human immunodeficiency virus seropositivity among children 1-24 months old in Kinshasa, Zaire. *Lancet* 1986: ii: 654-7.

[2] Lepage P, Van de Perre P, Carael, M. Are medical injections a risk factor for HIV infection in children? *Lancet* 1986; 328: 1103-1104.

[3] Lepage P, Van de Perre P. Nosocomial transmission of HIV in Africa: What tribute is paid to contaminated blood transfusions and medical injections? *Infect Cont Hosp Epidemiology* 1988; 9: 200-203.

[4] Quinn TC, Mann JM, Curran JW, Piot P. AIDS in Africa: an epidemiologic paradigm. *Science* 1986; 234: 955-963.

[5] Global Programme on AIDS. *1992-93 Progress Report: Global Programme on AIDS.* Geneva: WHO, 1995.

[6] WHO. *AIDS and HIV infection: information for United Nations employees and their families.* WHO/GPA/DIR/91.9. Geneva: WHO, 1991.

[7] WHO. Report of the Expanded Programme on Immunization, Global Advisory Group meeting, Washington DC, 9-13 November 1987. WHO/EPI/GEN/88.1. Geneva: WHO, 1988.

[8] WHO, UNICEF. Joint WHO/UNICEF statement on immunization and HIV/AIDS: the risk of transmitting HIV infection through immunization. *EPI newsletter: expanded program on immunization in the Americas* 1987; 9: 6-8.

[9] Berkley S, Weeks S, Barrenzi J. Immunization and fear of AIDS. *Lancet* 1990; i: 47-48.

[10] Davey S. *State of the world's vaccines and immunizations.* Geneva: WHO, 1996.

[11] Heymann DL, Piot P. The laboratory, epidemiology, nosocomial infection and HIV. *AIDS* 1994; 8: 705-706.

[12] WHO. Evaluation of injection technologies. WHO/EPI/CCIS/87.2. Geneva: WHO, 1987.

[13] Simonsen L, Kane A, Lloyd J, et al. Unsafe injections in the developing world and transmission of bloodborne pathogens: a review. *Bull World Health Organ* 1999; 77: 789-800.

[14] Kane A, Lloyd M, Zaffran M, et al. Transmission of hepatitis B, hepatitis C and human immunodeficiency viruses through unsafe injections in the developing world: Model-based regional estimates. *Bull World Health Organ* 1999; 77: 801-7.

[15] WHO, UNICEF, UNFPA. Safety of Injections: WHO-UNICEF-UNFPA joint statement on the use of auto-disable syringes in immunization services, 2nd rev. WHO/V&B/99.25. Geneva: WHO, 1999.

[16] Hutin YFJ, Hauri A, Armstrong GL. Use of injections in healthcare settings worldwide, 2000: literature review and regional estimates. *BMJ* 2003; 387: 1075.

[17] Hauri AM, Armstrong GL, Hutin YFJ. The global burden of disease attributable to contaminated injections given in health care settings. *Int J STD AIDS* 2004; 15: 7-16.

[18] Gisselquist D, Rothenberg R, Potterat JJ, Drucker E. HIV infections in sub-Sahara Africa not explained by sexual or vertical transmission. *Int J STD AIDS* 2002; 13: 657-666.

[19] Gisselquist D, Potterat JJ, Brody S, Vachon F. Let it be sexual: how health care transmission of AIDS in Africa was ignored. *Int J STD AIDS* 2003; 14: 148-161.

[20] Gisselquist D, Potterat JJ. Heterosexual transmission of HIV in Africa: an empiric estimate. *Int J STD AIDS* 2003; 14: 162-173.

[21] WHO. Unsafe injection practices and HIV infection: 14 March 2003, Geneva, WHO and UNAIDS. Geneva: WHO, 2003.

[22] Schmid GP, Buve A, Mugyenyi P, et al. Transmission of HIV-infection in sub-Saharan Africa and effect of elimination of unsafe injections. *Lancet* 2004; 363: 482-488.

[23] UNAIDS. *Living in a World with HIV and AIDS: Information for employees of the UN system and their families*, 1st rev. UNAIDS/04.27E. Geneva: UNAIDS, 2004.

[24] World Alliance for Patient Safety. *WHO draft guidelines for adverse event reporting and learning systems.* WHO/EIP/SPO/QPS/05.3. Geneva: WHO, 2005.

[25] Pepin J, Abou Chakra CN, Pepin E, et al. Evolution of the global use of unsafe medical injections, 2000-2010. *PLoS One* 2013; 8: e80948.

[26] Hayashi T, Hutin YJ-F, Bulterys M, et al. Injection practices in 2011-15: a review using data from the Demographic and Health Surveys (DHS). *BMC Health Serv Res* 2019; 19: 600.

[27] ICF. *République Démocratique du Congo: Evaluation des Prestations des Services de soins de Santé (EPSS RDC) 2017- 2018.* Rockville (MD): ICF, 2019.

[28] ICF Macro. *Kenya Service Provision Assessment Survey 2010.* Rockville (MD): ICF Macro, 2011.

[29] ICF International. *Malawi Service Provision Assessment (MSPA) 2013-14.* Rockville (MD): ICF International, 2014.

[30] ICF Macro. *Namibia Health Facility Census 2009.* Rockville (MD): ICF Macro, 2010.

[31] Macro International. *Rwanda Service Provision Assessment Survey 2007.* Calverton (MD): Macro International, 2008.

[32] ICF. *Sénégal: Enquête Continue sur la Prestation des Services de Soins de Santé (ECPSS) 2018.* Rockville (MD): ICF, 2020.

[33] ICF International. *Tanzania Service Provision Assessment Survey (TSPA) 2014-15.* Rockville (MD): ICF Internation, 2016.

[34] Macro International. *Uganda Service Provision Assessment Survey 2007.* Calverton (MD), Macro International, 2008.

[35] ORC Macro. *Zambia HIV/AIDS Service Provision Assessment Survey 2005.* Calverton (MD): ORC Macro, 2006.

[36] World Alliance for Patient Safety. *World Alliance for Patient Safety: forward program 2005.* Geneva: WHO, 2004.

[37] WHO. *WHO guideline on the use of safety-engineered syringes for intramuscular, intradermal, and subcutaneous injections in health-care settings.* Geneva: WHO, 2016.

[38] WHO. *Managing an injection safety policy.* Geneva: WHO, 2015.

[39] WHO. *Global health sector strategies on HIV, 2016-21.* Geneva: WHO, 2016.

[40] UNAIDS. *On the fast-track to end AIDS.* Geneva: UNAIDS, 2016.

[41] About. The Botswana-Harvard AIDS Institute Partnership [internet], 5 February 2018. Available at: https://bhp.org.bw/?page_id=11 (accessed 25 August 2020).

[42] Farmer P. Paul Farmer reports from Lesotho on the eve of the PIH project's first anniversary. Partners in Health [internet], 28 August 2007. Available at: https://www.pih.org/article/paul-farmer-reports-from-lesotho-on-the-eve-of-the-pih-projects-first (accessed 24 August 2020).

[43] World Medical Association (WMA). WMA Declaration of Lisbon on the Rights of the Patient, revised 2005, reaffirmed 2015. Ferney-Voltaire: WMA, 2015.

[44] WHO. Constitution of the World Health Organization, in: *Basic documents*, 45th ed, suppl. Geneva: WHO, 2006.

[45] Gisselquist D, Friedman E, Potterat J, et al. Four policies to reduce HIV transmission through unsterile health care. *Int J STD AIDS* 2003; 14: 717-722.

[46] Gisselquist D, Potterat JJ, St Lawrence JS, et al. How to contain generalized epidemics: a plea for better evidence to displace speculation. *Int J STD AIDS* 2009; 20: 443-446.

CHAPTER FOUR

African Governments Accept Unexplained HIV Infections

Outside of sub-Saharan Africa, the general public, media, and government have characteristically shown a low tolerance for unexplained HIV infections in the general population. Such sentiments are not evident in Africa.

As described here, unexplained infections reported in sub-Saharan Africa are far more common than unexplained infections that launched outbreak investigations in other countries around the world. Yet there have been no similar investigations – identifying suspected source facilities then testing others treated at those facilities – anywhere in sub-Sahara Africa.

South Africa gets special attention. Despite the country's economic strength and scientific abilities, government has sat on the sidelines, watching the development of one of the world's worst HIV epidemics.

The last section of this chapter speculates about why governments have not investigated.

Unexplained infections in national surveys

Most governments in sub-Saharan Africa have tested adults for HIV in random sample national surveys, and some have tested children as well. In the latest national surveys from all countries with at least 5% of adults HIV-positive, the percentage of self-declared virgins aged 15-24 years who tested HIV-positive ranged as high as 6.3% for men and 5.0% for women (Figure 4.1).

In seven national surveys that tested mothers and children for HIV, the percentage of HIV-positive children with mothers who test HIV-negative ranged from 6% to 33% (Figure 4.2). The child-mother pairs tested in surveys likely include many mothers who had gotten HIV from their children. If children were still breastfeeding when they got HIV from health care, evidence from investigated outbreaks suggests 40%-60% would infect their mothers[16] (see also Chapter 2). In Mozambique, for example, it is likely that more than 50% of HIV-positive children aged 6-23 months in the 2015 survey got HIV from health care, and that many had infected their mothers before the survey.

Figure 4.1: Percentages of self-reported virgin men and women aged 15-24 years who tested HIV-positive in national surveys

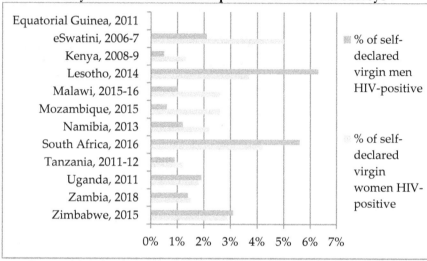

Sources: Equatorial Guinea[1]; eSwatini[2]; Kenya[3]; Lesotho[4]; Malawi[5]; Mozambique[6]; Namibia[7]; South Africa[8]; Tanzania[9]; Uganda[10]; Zambia[#26 in Chapter 6]; Zimbabwe.[11]

Figure 4.2: Percentages* of HIV-positive children with HIV-negative mothers from national surveys

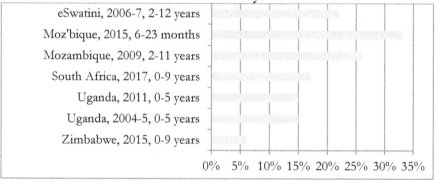

*Percentages for Mozambique, Uganda, and Zimbabwe are estimated from reported numbers of mothers infected, not infected, or not tested and percentages of children HIV-positive according to the mother's HIV status. For eSwatini and South Africa, the figure shows the percentages of HIV-positive children with HIV-negative mothers for children with tested mothers only.
Sources: eSwatini[12]; Mozambique[6,13]; South Africa[14]; Uganda[10,15]; Zimbabwe.[11]

In at least one instance, reports of children with unexplained HIV got the attention of local media. After newspapers in eSwatini reported findings from the country's 2006-7 survey that 22% of HIV-positive children aged 2-12 years had HIV-negative mothers (among children with tested mothers), a newspaper editorial and a senator asked the minister of health to set up a commission to look into the matter.[17] As far as I know, nothing was done. Doctors from United Kingdom and US criticized that public discussion of the possibility that health care had infected children had "detrimentally affected both health-care provision and research in Swaziland."[18]

High rates of new HIV infections in pregnant women

Women have been on the front lines for HIV tests. To prevent mother-to-child HIV transmission, most pregnant women in Africa get tested for HIV. Because women with new infections are at high risk to infect their babies, researchers have paid a lot of attention to the rates at which pregnant and breastfeeding women get HIV. This has led to dozens of studies that have found and reported those rates.[19] A typical study tests women for HIV at their first antenatal visit, then tests them again when they deliver.

Many such studies report pregnant women in specific hospitals and clinics getting new HIV infections at high rates. For example, in eight large studies (reporting more than 20 new infections each) in five countries, pregnant women and new mothers got HIV at rates ranging from 6.8% to 19% per year (Table 4.1). If women got HIV at such rates through 2-3 pregnancies, the percentage of women HIV-positive would be greater than for all adults in the country (see last column on the right in Table 4.1).

Rather than considering the possibility that at least some women were getting HIV from unsafe health care, all study teams assumed (without testing and tracing husbands) that all new infections came from sex. That is not likely, considering: (a) the percentage of adults infected in the country (right column in Table 4.1) gives a rough idea about the percentage of husbands infected; (b) only a small fraction of infected husbands transmit HIV in a year (Table A2.1); and (c) some infected husbands would have already infected their wives before the observed pregnancy.

Not testing husbands to see if they might have infected their wives was not only bad science, it was also not taking care of either him or the family. When a wife has a new infection, but the husband is HIV-negative, that should be recognized, and the couple should be warned to protect him and thereby the family's and children's future.

Table 4.1: New HIV infections in women during pregnancy and after delivery*

Country, year	New HIV infections in pregnant women			% of adults in the country HIV-positive during study years
	Rate women got HIV (%/year)	Study sites	When did women get HIV?	
eSwatini, 2004, 2006[21]	19.0%†	17 clinics	6 months before ANC	25.3%
eSwatini, 2008-9[22]	16.8%	6 clinics	ANC to delivery	27.0%
Zimbabwe, 1990-93[23]	13.3%†	4 clinics	ANC to 6 months PP	19.5%
South Africa, 2011-12[24]	11.2%†	580 clinics	ANC to delivery	18.7%
South Africa, 2002-5[25]	11.0%†	3 studies	during pregnancy	15.5%
South Africa, 2006-7[26]	10.7%	9 clinics	ANC to later ANC	17.0%
Malawi, 1990-4[27]	7.99%	1 hospital	ANC to delivery	10.5%
Kenya, 2008[28]	6.8%	6 clinics	ANC to 6 weeks PP	6.6%

Abbreviations: ANC: antenatal care; PP: post-partum. *All studies reporting women getting HIV at rates of at least 6% per year and with at least 20 new infections. †These percentages are calculated from information reported by each study, as explained in a recent review.[19]

Sources: For HIV infections in women, see references in each row; a recent review[19] describes the study search. Percentage of adults HIV-positive in the country during study years are from UNAIDS.[20]

Studies in Table 4.1 represent missed opportunities for governments to identify unexplained infections and to find and fix unsafe health care. Pregnant women have a lot of potential exposures to HIV-contaminated blood (such as blood tests, tetanus vaccinations, and delivery). High rates of new infections reported in Table 4.1 should have alerted public health officials that pregnancy-related health care may be infecting women. Opportunities to find and to investigate unexplained infections continue with routine testing of pregnant women to prevent mother-to-child HIV transmission.

Women may get HIV from health care not only directly but also indirectly through their babies. Babies infected from health care may infect mothers through breastfeeding, as seen in Russia, Libya, and elsewhere (Chapter 2). This has not been reported in Africa, but there is some evidence. A study in Rwanda that followed HIV-negative child-mother pairs during 1989-94 recognized new infections in one mother-baby pair at the same time, six months after delivery. After sequencing multiple HIVs from both the baby and the mother, researchers found more diversity in the baby's HIV than in the mother's. More diversity in the baby's HIV suggests the baby was infected first.[29]

Sentinel surveys

Women have been on the front lines for HIV tests for many years. In the late 1980s, most African governments began "sentinel surveys" of pregnant women attending various antenatal clinics to monitor what was happening with the countries' HIV epidemics. Sentinel surveys took blood collected for other purposes and removed women's names before testing, so neither the women nor anyone else knew who was infected.

Some of the extremely high percentages of HIV-positive pregnant women reported from sentinel surveys should have rung alarm bells. For example, in 1994 and again in 2000, more than 70% of pregnant women tested HIV-positive in sentinel surveys at an antenatal clinic in Chiredzi in southeast Zimbabwe.[30] In Botswana, sentinel surveys reported more than 50% of antenatal women were HIV-positive at three sites in one or more years during 1999-2002.[31] These percentages not only document human tragedies, they also represent missed opportunities to protect women.

Studies find bunches of unexplained infections

Over the years, hundreds of studies across Africa have tested selected populations for HIV infections. Many such studies have reported unexplained infections in children with HIV-negative mothers and in adult and adolescent men and women reporting no sexual risks. When a government is ready to investigate unexplained infections, such studies show good places to start. Chapter 3 reports several studies that found unexplained infections in children. Here are a few more examples for children and adults.

South Sudan, 2018

Ten of 24 HIV-positive children aged 0-14 years at Al Sabah Children's Hospital in Juba, South Sudan, had HIV-negative mothers. The article reporting these infections says nothing about how the 10 children might have gotten HIV.[32]

Nigeria, 2010

Among children aged two months to 15 years seeking health care in Kano, 22 tested HIV-positive. For five children, the study team identified the probable mode of transmission as group circumcision.[33]

Botswana, 2000-4

Among adults attending 16 voluntary testing and counseling sites, 136 (4.2%) of 3,274 self-reported virgins were HIV-positive.[34]

Zimbabwe, 1998-2003

To study risks for HIV infection in Manicaland, researchers tested adult men and women during 1998-2000, then retested them three years later, in 2001-3. Nineteen women and eight men who reported no sex partners over three years got HIV.[35] Adults reporting no sex partners over three years got HIV at the rate of 1.1% per year (compared to 1.9% for adults reporting one or more sex partners) and accounted for 13% of observed new infections.

South Africa's failure to investigate

South Africa, where doctors achieved the first human heart transplant and one of the wealthiest countries in Africa, has a terrible HIV epidemic. In 2015, an estimated 30.8% of pregnant women were HIV-positive at antenatal clinics throughout South Africa, with more pregnant women infected in parts of the country: for example, 44.5% in KwaZulu-

Natal province and 48.4% in Zululand district of that province[36] (see also Figure A1.3). Even more adults were infected in some age cohorts and regions. For example, in a 2014 survey in a region of uMungundlovu district, KwaZulu-Natal, 66.4% of women aged 35-39 years were HIV-positive as were 59.6% of men aged 40-44 years.[37] Although South Africa has only 0.75% of the world's population, UNAIDS estimates 7.5 million South Africans were HIV-positive in 2019,[20] almost a fifth of the world's total HIV infections (a 2017 national survey estimated 7.9 million infected[14]).

Over the years, surveys, researchers, and media have recognized and reported unexplained HIV infections. As of mid-2020, government had not investigated any such infection by identifying facilities that might have infected patients and inviting others treated at those facilities to come for tests. For example, beginning in 1999, a group of doctors in Cape Town from time to time recognized 30 HIV-positive children with HIV-negative mothers and asked about and reported healthcare events that might have infected them.[38-40] But government has not subsequently traced and tested others treated at suspected source facilities to see if the facilities had infected others and to find and fix errors.

A lot of evidence suggests HIV transmission through skin-piercing procedures in health care, and possibly also during cosmetic services, has been and remains common in South Africa. Following subsections summarize selected evidence from later to earlier observations.

2011-17: 82 unexplained infections in young women in Mpumalanga

A 2011-12 study in Mpumalanga province tested 2,533 high school women aged 13-20 years; 81 were HIV-positive, including 38 who reported never having vaginal or anal sex.[41] The study then followed and retested the women for 1-6 years, during which time 190 got HIV, including 44 who reported no lifetime sex.[42]

2014-15: 207 unexplained HIV infections in KwaZulu-Natal

A 2014-15 survey among adults aged 15-49 years in parts of uMgungundlovu district, KwaZulu-Natal, found 207 with unexplained

HIV infections, including 137 (11.2% of 818) self-reported virgin women and 70 (9.0% of 692) virgin men.[37]

2013-14: Cluster of 63 recent infections in KwaZulu-Natal

A study that collected blood from a random sample of adults in parts of uMkhanyakude district, KwaZulu-Natal, found evidence of a large HIV outbreak best explained by bloodborne transmission.[43] I present and discuss this evidence along with experts' and government's responses in Chapter 5.

2012: 77 unexplained infections in high school students in KwaZulu-Natal

In a 2012 survey among students in grades 8-12, averaging 15.8 years old, in KwaZulu-Natal, 56 (54%) of 104 HIV-positive girls and 21 (55%) of 38 HIV-positive boys said they had never had sex.[44]

2005: National survey reported unexplained new HIV infections

South Africa's 2005 national HIV survey used blood tests to distinguish new HIV infections from old ones. From such tests, the survey estimated that: children aged 2-14 years got HIV at the rate of 0.5% per year; self-reported virgin adults got new infections at the rate of 1.5% per year; adults who were sexually active in the previous year got HIV at 2.4% per year; and non-virgin adults who reported no sex partner in the previous year got HIV at the same 2.4% annual rate.[45]

2005: National survey reports people who got more health care from public vs. private services were more likely to be HIV-positive

South Africa's 2005 national HIV survey reported a much higher percentage of Black Africans aged two years and older was HIV-positive (13.3%) compared to Whites (0.6%). These differences parallel differences in where people get health care: 84.2% of Black Africans aged 15 years and older said they got most health care from public services while 80.8% of Whites reported they got most health care from private providers.[46]

1986-94: South Africa's early epidemic doubled every 9-13 months

During 1986-90, the estimated number of infections in Black Africans doubled roughly every nine months.[47] During 1990-94, the doubling time for numbers of infections in pregnant women throughout South Africa averaged 13 months (from 0.7% in 1990 to 7.6% of a larger population in 1994).[36] Such rapid increases in numbers of infections should have raised eyebrows, alerting people that more than sex was involved. The speed of HIV transmission required for such rapid epidemic expansion was much faster than the 9% per year rate of sexual transmission observed as early as 1990-91 in Africa in a study that followed HIV-negative adults with HIV-positive husbands or wives in Uganda (see Table A2.1).

Good things happening, but something missing

The South African government is doing a lot of what is required to respond to this epidemic. With more testing, anti-retroviral treatment (ART), and programs to prevent mother-to-child transmission, estimated AIDS deaths among all ages fell by three-fourths from 290,000 in 2006 to 72,000 in 2019. The estimated annual number of new HIV infections fell as well, but not as fast: from 550,000 in 2001 to 200,000 in 2019.[20] South Africa's HIV/AIDS disaster has been reaching the next generation. In 2017 young women aged 15-24 years were getting HIV at the rate of 1.51% per year.[14]

Along with all the good things that are happening, something is missing. When will communities and government in South Africa investigate to protect public health?

Why do governments not investigate?

Public health managers in Africa have been aware that health care facilities reuse skin-piercing instruments. In 1994, for example, Africa's ministers of health endorsed the Yamoussoukro declaration: that 95% of injections for immunization should use sterile syringes and needles by 1997.[48] By not asking for 100% of injections with sterile equipment, the ministers acknowledged injections were unreliably sterile.

Many African scientists recognize the contribution of bloodborne transmission to Africa's HIV epidemics. For example, a 2002-4 study reported by Munyaradze Mapingure and colleagues found 25.6% of pregnant women to be HIV-positive in several clinics in Harare, Zimbabwe, compared to only 5.6% in Moshi, Tanzania.[49] Higher risk for women in Zimbabwe vs. Tanzania "cannot be explained by differences in risky sexual behaviour: all risk factors tested for in our study were higher for Tanzania than Zimbabwe. Non-sexual transmission of HIV might have played an important role in variation of HIV prevalence."

Similarly, health officials and experts in Africa have investigated and reported hospitals transmitting other diseases. For example, experts traced an outbreak of extensively drug-resistant (XDR) tuberculosis in KwaZulu-Natal, South Africa, to one hospital.[50] The investigation showed that already infected and susceptible patients had been in the same hospital ward at the same time during 2005-6 and sequenced their tuberculosis samples to show their infections were linked.

Despite awareness of bloodborne risks for HIV and demonstrated willingness to investigate a hospital-based tuberculosis outbreak in South Africa, no ministry of health across sub-Saharan Africa has similarly investigated any unexplained HIV infection to find linked infections and to find and fix their source.

Domestic considerations and foreign influence

Public trust is important for public health programs. Governments may foster public trust by assuring people they have little or no risk to get HIV from health care, even if that is not so. Investigations would alert the public to risks, but at the same time find and fix risks, so that future assurances could be based on reality. Without investigations, some officials may genuinely think risks are small, or that health care is so important that risks can be overlooked. But even when public health managers know that investigating is the right thing to do, they may not want to face public awareness of risks, public criticism, and public pressure for healthcare programs to be more accountable to patients.

Foreign money and experts have a lot of influence on healthcare policies and programs in Africa.[51] International and foreign organizations have advised Africans to expect unknown numbers of HIV infections from health care (see Chapter 3). How and to what extent foreign aid and advice influence government decisions is something the people involved might not want to talk about. How much aid money and job opportunities are predicated on doing what donors want? How much are local experts and officials swayed by foreign experts and publications expounding unsupported theories about Africa's epidemics?

Whatever has been the mechanism for foreign influence, the outcome seems clear: Governments that get little or no HIV/AIDS money from the international community, including governments of Pakistan, Cambodia, Kazakhstan, Kyrgyzstan, Libya, and Uzbekistan, have investigated outbreaks, whereas governments in sub-Saharan Africa that get most such aid have not.

Getting to yes

Why have government officials in sub-Saharan Africa consistently decided not to investigate? Whatever the mix of reasons might be in any specific situation, for people at risk who want government help to investigate unexplained HIV infections in their communities, the challenge is the same: to get officials to push aside those reasons and to do what is needed to protect public health.

References

[1] ICF International. *Guinea Ecuatorial Encuesta Demográfica y de Salud (EDSGE-I) 2011*. Rockville (MD): ICF International, 2012.

[2] Macro International. *Swaziland Demographic and Health Survey 2006-07*. Calverton (MD): Macro International, 2008.

[3] ICF Macro. *Kenya Demographic and Health Survey 2008-09*. Rockville (MD): ICF Macro, 2010.

[4] ICF International. *Lesotho Demographic and Health Survey 2014*. Rockville (MD): ICF International, 2016.

[5] ICF. *Malawi Demographic and Health Survey 2015-16*. Rockville (MD): ICF, 2017.

[6] ICF. *Inquérito de Indicadores de Imunização, Malária e HIV/SIDA em Moçambique 2015*. Rockville (MD): ICF, 2018.

[7] ICF International. *The Namibia Demographic and Health Survey 2013*. Rockville (MD): ICF International, 2014.

[8] ICF. *South Africa Demographic and Health Survey 2016*. Pretoria, South Africa, and Rockville (MD): ICF, 2019.

[9] ICF International. *Tanzania HIV/AIDS and Malaria Indicator Survey 2011-12.* Rockville (MD): ICF International, 2013.

[10] ICF International. *Uganda AIDS Indicator Survey 2011.* Rockville (MD): ICF International, 2012.

[11] ICF International. *Zimbabwe Demographic and Health Survey 2015: Final Report.* Rockville (MD): ICF International, 2016.

[12] Okinyi M, Brewer DD, Potterat JJ. Horizontally acquired HIV infection in Kenyan and Swazi children. *Int J STD AIDS* 2009; 20: 852-857.

[13] ICF Macro. *Inquérito Nacional de Prevalência, Riscos Comportamentais e Informação sobre o HIV e SIDA em Moçambique 2009.* Calverton (MD): ICF Macro, 2010.

[14] Simbayi LC, Zuma K, Zungu N, et al. *South African National HIV Prevalence, Incidence, Behaviour and Communications Survey 2017.* Cape Town: Human Sciences Research Council; 2019.

[15] ORC Macro. *Uganda HIV/AIDS Sero-Behavioural Survey 2004-05.* Calverton (MD): ORC Macro, 2006.

[16] Little KM, Kilmarx PH, Taylor AW, et al. A review of evidence for transmission of HIV from children to breastfeeding women and implications for prevention. *Pediatr Infect Dis J* 2012; 31: 938-942.

[17] Rooney R. No room for Swaziland HIV denial. *Swaziland Media Commentary* 3 December 2009.

[18] Adler MR, Church K. Limitations and implications of generalizations made regarding horizontal HIV transmission in Swaziland. *Int J STD AIDS* 2011; 22: 117-120.

[19] Gisselquist D. Missed signals: not investigating high HIV incidence in pregnant women in Africa. *Social Science Research Network* [internet] 17 April 2018. Available at: https://papers.ssrn.com/sol3/papers.cfm?abstract_id=3153795 (accessed 16 June 2020).

[20] UNAIDS. HIV estimates with uncertainty bounds 1990-2019. Geneva: UNAIDS, 2020.

[21] Bernasconi D, Tavoschi L, Regine V, et al. Identification of recent HIV infections and of factors associated with virus acquisition among pregnant women in 2004 and 2006 in Swaziland. *J Clin Virol* 2010; 48: 180-183.

[22] Kieffer MP, Nhlabatsi B, Mahdi M, et al. Improved detection of incident HIV infection and uptake of PMTCT services in labor and delivery in a high HIV prevalence setting. *J Acquir Immune Defic Syndr* 2011; 57: e85-e91.

23 Mbizvo MT, Kasule J, Mahomed K, et al. HIV-1 seroconversion incidence following pregnancy and delivery among women seronegative at recruitment in Harare, Zimbabwe. *Cent Afr J Med* 2001; 47: 115-118.

24 Dinh T-H, Delaney KP, Goga A, et al. Impact of maternal HIV seroconversion during pregnancy on early mother to child transission of HIV (MTCT) measured at 4-8 weeks postpartum in South Africa 2011-2012: a national population-base survey. *PLoS* 2015; 10: e0125525.

25 Wand H, Ramjee G. Combined impact of sexual risk behaviors for HIV seroconversion among women in Durban, South Africa: implications for prevention policy and planning. *AIDS Behav* 2011; 15: 479-486.

26 Moodley D, Esterhuizen TM, Pather T, et al. High HIV incidence during pregnancy: compelling reason for repeat testing. *AIDS* 2009; 23: 1255-1259.

27 Taha TE, Hoover DR, Dallabetta GA, et al. Bacterial vaginosis and disturbances of vaginal flora: association with increased acquisition of HIV. *AIDS* 1998; 12: 1669-1706.

28 Kinuthia J, Kiarie JN, Farquhar C, et al. Cofactors for HIV-1 incidence during pregnancy and postpartum period. *Curr HIV Res* 2010; 8: 510-514.

29 Kampinga GA, Simonon A, Van de Perre P, et al. Primary infections with HIV-1 women and their offspring in Rwanda: findings heterogeneity at seroconversion, coinfection, and recombinants of HIV-1 subtypes A and C. *Virol* 1997; 227: 63-76.

30 UNAIDS. Zimbabwe: epidemiological fact sheets on HIV/AIDS and sexually transmitted infections, 2002 update. Geneva: UNAIDS, 2002.

31 UNAIDS. Botswana: epidemiological fact sheets on HIV/AIDS and sexually transmitted infections, 2004 update. Geneva: UNAIDS, 2004.

32 Gel G, Kitaka SB, Musiime V, et al. Prevalence, clinical pattern and immediate outcomes of HIV-infected children admitted to Al Sabah Children's Hospital, South Sudan. *So Sudan Med J* 2019; 12: 85-88.

33 Obiagwu PN, Hassan-Hanga F, Ibrahim M. Pediatric HIV in Kano, Nigeria. *Nigerian J Clin Practice* 2013; 16: 521-525.

34 Creek T, Alwano MG, Molosiwa RR, et al. Botswana's Tebelopele voluntary HIV counseling and testing network: use and client risk

factors for HIV infection, 2000-2004. *J Acquir Immune Defic Syndr* 2006; 43: 210-218.

[35] Lopman B, Nyamukapa C, Mushati P, et al. HIV incidence in 3 years of follow-up of a Zimbabwe cohort – 1998-2000 to 2001-03: contributions to proximate and underlying determinants to transmission. *Int J Epidemiol* 2008; 37: 88-103.

[36] National Department of Health (NDoH). *The 2015 National Antenatal Sentinel HIV & Syphilis Survey, South Africa.* Pretoria: NDoH, 2017.

[37] Kharsany ABM, Cawood C, Khanyile D, et al. Community-based HIV prevalence in KwaZulu-Natal, South Africa: results of a cross-sectional household survey. *Lancet HIV* 2018; 5: e 427-e437.

[38] Hiemstra R, Rabie H, Schaaf HS, et al. Unexplained HIV-1 infections in children – documenting cases and assessing for possible risk factors. *S Afr Med J* 2004; 94: 188-193.

[39] Slogrove S, Rabie H, Cotton M. Non-vertical transmission of HIV in children: more evidence from the Western Cape, South Africa. *VI Int AIDS Soc Conf HIV Path Treat Prevent*, Rome, July 2011. Abstract CDC137.

[40] Myburgh D, Rabie H, Slogrove AL, et al. Horizontal HIV transmission to children of HIV-uninfected mothers: a case series and review of the global literature. *Int J Infect Dis* 2020; 98: 315-320.

[41] Pettifor A, MacPhail C, Selin A, et al. HPTN 068: a randomized control trial of a conditional cash transfer to reduce HIV infection in young women in South Africa – study design and baseline results. *AIDS Behav* 2016; 9: 1863-1882.

[42] Stoner MCD, Nguyen N, Kilburn K, et al. Age-disparate partnerships and incident HIV infection in adolescent girls and young women in rural South Africa. *AIDS* 2019; 33: 83-91.

[43] Coltart C, Shahmanesh M, Hue S, et al. Ongoing HIV micro-epidemics in rural South Africa: the need for flexible interventions. *Conference on Retroviruses and Opportunistic Infections*, Boston 4-7 March 2018. Abstract 47LB and oral presentation.

[44] Kharsany ABM, Buthelezi TJ, Frohlich JA, et al. HIV infection in high school students in rural South Africa: role of transmissions among students. *AIDS Res Hum Retroviruses* 2014; 30: 956-965.

[45] Rehle T, Shisana O, Pillay V, et al. National HIV incidence measures – new insights into the South African epidemic. *S Afr Med J* 2007; 97: 194-199.

[46] Shisana O, Rehle T, Simbayi L, et al. *South African National HIV Prevalence, Incidence, Behavior and Communication Survey, 2005*. Cape Town: Human Sciences Research Council, 2005.

[47] Padayachee GN, Schall R. Short-term predictions of the prevalence of human immunodeficiency virus infection among the black population in South Africa. *S Afr Med J* 1990; 77: 329-323.

[48] Davey S, *State of the world's vaccines and immunization*. Geneva: WHO, 1996.

[49] Mapingure MP, Msuya S, Kurewa NE, et al. Sexual behavior does not reflect HIV-1 prevalence differences: a comparison study of Zimbabwe and Tanzania. *J Int AIDS Soc* 2010; 13: 45.

[50] Ghandi NR, Weissman D, Woodley P, et al. Nosocomial transmission of extensively drug-resistant tuberculosis in a rural hospital in South Africa. *J Infect Dis* 2013; 207: 9-17.

[51] Hunsmann M. *Depoliticising an epidemic -- International AIDS control and the politics of health in Tanzania*. PhD dissertation. Freiburg: Albert-Ludwigs-Universitat, 2013.

CHAPTER FIVE

Evidence from a Double-barreled Smoking Gun[1]

> The term "smoking gun" is a reference to an object or fact that serves as conclusive evidence of a crime or similar act...[2]

A recent double-barreled smoking gun calls attention to long-term mistakes that have left Africans at risk to get HIV from health care. The first smoking barrel was the discovery of a large HIV outbreak in South Africa in 2013-14 that is best explained by bloodborne transmission, most likely during health care. The second smoking barrel is the subsequent silence by public health and HIV/AIDS officials and experts about the likelihood that unsafe health care caused the outbreak.

First smoking barrel: evidence of HIV from health care in Kwazulu-Natal, 2013-14

In 2010-14, researchers collected HIV from a random sample of adults in a large mostly rural study area in uMkhanyakude district in KwaZulu-Natal. The team then sequenced 1,376 HIV samples (i.e., determined the order of HIV's component parts). Because HIV changes over time, similar sequences from two or more people suggest recent and close transmission links. Among the 1,376 sequences, the study team found a cluster of 63 very similar HIV. The study estimated that HIV from one person in June 2013 had somehow reached and infected 63 people within 18 months through November 2014.[3]

Because the 1,376 HIV sequences came from an estimated 9% of HIV-positive adults in the study area, the observed cluster of 63 similar HIV may well be 9% of a much larger cluster of 600-800 closely linked infections in the study area. Moreover, because many of the 63 similar HIV came from people living in a town on the border of the study area, the cluster likely extends outside the area. And transmission appeared to be ongoing when the study stopped collecting HIV samples in 2014.

In their conference presentation, the study team showed a "tree" diagram linking the 63 similar sequences to an estimated parent virus in mid-2013 (slide 10 in[3]). This tree, showing rapid and recent transmission links, is similar to a tree linking HIV sequences from the investigated outbreak from unsafe health care discovered in Roka, Cambodia in 2014 (Figure 2b in[4]).

The study that reported the 2013-14 outbreak in KwaZulu-Natal suggested HIV might have spread through sex, but provides no information about sexual risks for anyone in the cluster. In any case, the possibility that sex could transmit HIV from 1 to 63 infections (much less hundreds) in 18 months is vanishingly small, considering:

- Sexual transmission is far too slow. Even between spouses, it takes on average years for one to infect the other. Combining data from five studies in Africa in which many or most spouses did not know one was infected, HIV-negative partners got new HIV infections at a rate of less than 10% per year (Table A2.1). In a 2016 national survey in South Africa, in couples with at least one partner HIV-positive, less than half of their partners were infected.[5]
- According to self-reported sexual behavior, having multiple partners had little to do with HIV transmission in the study area. Repeat surveys in the study area during 2004-15 identified 2,367 new HIV infections in adults. Only 43 (1.8%) of 2,367 adults with new infections reported more than one sex partner in the previous year, while 189 (8.0%) of 2,367 adults with new infections said they were virgins (Table 1 in[6]).

Second smoking barrel: expert and official silence about the likelihood health care infected patients

Researchers from the African Health Research Institute and the University College London collected HIV from the study area in 2010-14 and then sequenced HIV samples and discovered the cluster of 63 infections in 2017. They reported their discovery in March 2018 at the Conference on Retroviruses and Opportunistic Infections in Boston.

Because it is almost impossible for such an outbreak to come from anything other than bloodborne transmission, the government of South Africa could protect public health by investigating to find and fix whatever caused it. Investigators should ask people in the cluster what skin-piercing procedures they received and where during 2013-14, and then invite others who visited suspected facilities to come for HIV tests.

Even if someone wants to argue or believe that sex could somehow account for all infections in the cluster, bloodborne transmission remains a possible explanation. That possibility challenges the government to investigate. We[1] have found no evidence the government of South Africa has taken any steps to investigate that possibility.

During their 2018 Conference presentation, the research team did not acknowledge the possibility unsafe health care caused the outbreak, and none of the discussants mentioned such risks. To the best of our knowledge, as we are writing this more than two years after the cluster was reported in 2018, no expert in gene sequencing and no HIV expert or official in any international or foreign organization has acknowledged the possibility the cluster comes from unsafe health care.

Considering the many experts who are aware of the cluster, continuing silence about what is so obvious – that the cluster likely (or at least possibly) comes from unsafe health care – shows that people who understand the implications of the cluster are choosing to keep silent. That in turn suggests they are aware of pressures not to say what is obvious. Their silence is strong circumstantial evidence – smoking gun evidence – that officials who control research funds and jobs for people working on HIV do not want them to say that bloodborne risks very likely or even possibly caused the outbreak.

This has been going on for a long time!

Silence about the likelihood the large cluster of 63 closely linked infections in KwaZulu-Natal came from bloodborne risks is a recent example of more than three decades of inadequate responses to evidence of HIV from health care in Africa (Chapters 3 and 4).[7] Those who are silent include many experts in gene sequencing who have only recently started to look at HIV from Africa. Gene sequencing experts coming new to Africa's HIV epidemics have not been implicated in decades of inadequate responses to unexplained HIV infections. But now they, too, are silent.

Those who are silent are not explaining why. Because people are at risk, speculating about why experts and officials are not doing their jobs is a distraction. Setting aside distractions, the tasks at hand are: to get investigations underway to find and fix skin-piercing procedures that infect people; and to warn people about risks to get HIV from health care as long as those risks are not found and fixed.

References

[1] Simon Collery co-authored this chapter. See also: Gisselquist D, Collery S. Africa's HIV epidemics: Evidence from a double-barreled smoking gun. *Social Science Research Network* [internet] 1 May 2020. Available at: https://papers.ssrn.com/sol3/papers.cfm?abstract_id=3590251 (accessed 1 May 2020).

[2] Smoking gun. *Wikipedia* [internet] 29 April 2020. Available at: https://en.wikipedia.org/wiki/Smoking_gun (accessed 23 August 2020).

[3] Coltart CEM, Shahmanesh M, Hue S, et al. Ongoing HIV micro-epidemics in rural South Africa: the need for flexible interventions. *Conference on Retroviruses and Opportunistic Infections*, Boston, 4-7 March 2018. Abstract 47LB and oral abstract.

[4] Rouet F, Nouhin J, Zheng D-P, et al. Massive iatrogenic outbreak of human immunodeficiency virus type 1 in rural Cambodia, 2014-2015. *Clin Infect Dis* 2018; 66: 1733-1741.

[5] ICF. *South Africa Demographic and Health Survey 2016*. Rockville (MD): ICF, 2019.

[6] Akullian A Bershteyn A, Klein D, et al. Sexual partnership age pairings and risk of HIV acquisition in rural South Africa. *AIDS* 2017; 31: 1755-1764.

[7] Fernando D. The AIDS pandemic: searching for a global response. *J Assoc Nurses AIDS Care* 2018; 29: 635-641.

CHAPTER SIX

Rejecting the Myth that Almost All HIV Comes from Sex

Pervasive public health messages warning about HIV from sex can make it hard for people who know of one or more unexplained infections to get neighbors, reporters, clergy, and others to believe the infections did not come from sex, and that their source should be investigated. This chapter provides evidence and references that anyone can use to challenge the widely believed myth that sexual transmission accounts for almost all HIV infections among adults in Africa.

As reviewed here, the best evidence indicates that far less than half of HIV infections in Africa come from sex. Of course, sex is a risk for HIV, but that says nothing about how much comes from sex. Similarly, getting hit by a car is a risk, but that does not mean cars kill everyone. In both cases, people should take care to protect themselves even if the risk in question accounts for a minority of infections or deaths.

How the myth got started

Racial stereotypes of sexual behavior played a major role in early speculation about Africa's HIV epidemics, even within medical journals. For example, a 1986 editorial in the *Journal of the Royal Society of Medicine* attributed differences between HIV epidemics in the US and Europe vs. Africa to "the much lower contact rate... among North American and European heterosexuals."[1] A 1987 paper in the *Review of Epidemiology* states: "[M]ost traditional African societies are promiscuous by Western standards. Promiscuity occurs both premaritally and postmaritally" and "seems to be the most important cultural factor contributing to the transmission of HIV in Africa."[2] In 1988, the head of WHO's Global Programme on AIDS along with the future head of UNAIDS and others authored an article in *Science* claiming: "[S]tudies in Africa have demonstrated that HIV-1 is primarily a sexually transmitted disease and that the main risk factor for acquisition is the degree of sexual activity with multiple partners, not sexual orientation."[3]

In 1988, WHO experts estimated, without presenting any supporting evidence, that roughly 90% of HIV infections in adults in Africa came from heterosexual sex.[4] That estimate disagreed with evidence. As of 1988, the substantial amount of evidence already available about risks for HIV infections in Africa suggested bloodborne risks may have been causing more infections than sex.[5] That evidence includes: children with unexplained infections, both new and old HIV infections more common in people with recent medical injections, and infections not concentrated in sexually more active adults.

Soon after international experts committed to the myth, information from surveys about sexual behavior in countries around the world disagreed with racial stereotypes. A 2006 summary of information from such surveys reported a "comparatively high prevalence of multiple partnerships in developed countries, compared with parts of the world with far higher rates of sexually transmitted infections and HIV, such as African countries..."[6] Nevertheless, the myth lives on. Many people continue to think that differences in sexual behavior in Africa vs. the rest of the world explain Africa's HIV epidemics.

15 experts can't find evidence linking most HIV to sexual risks

During 2002-3, articles in medical journals along with presentations at a closed-door meeting at WHO challenged the idea that sex accounts for almost all HIV in Africa (see Chapter 3). In response, WHO and UNAIDS staff led a team of 15 authors publishing a rebuttal in *The Lancet* medical journal in 2004. The authors claimed: "epidemiological evidence indicates that sexual transmission continues to be by far the major mode of spread of HIV-1 in the [Africa] region."[7]

What evidence? The only evidence they presented linking HIV to sexual behavior was the age distribution of HIV-positive Africans: "the prevalence [percent infected] in children aged 5-14 years... was much lower than the prevalence in adolescents and adults aged 15 years or older." Women, especially, get more HIV infections beginning in their late teens. But does that show HIV comes from sex? Other risks change with age. From their late teens, women get more blood exposures from reproduction-related health care and maybe also from cosmetic services.

If the ages of those who get HIV is sufficient to show infections come from sex, then by that same argument, tuberculosis and even parking tickets are sexually transmitted.

The meager evidence presented to link HIV to sexual behavior is telling. The 15 authors had between them been involved in dozens of studies in Africa looking at sexual behavior as a risk for HIV infection. The problem for the 15 authors was that the huge body of available evidence on sexual behavior vs. HIV infection disagreed with their claim – adults reporting no partner, one HIV-negative partner, or 100% condom use were getting HIV.[8] As an excuse for ignoring disagreeable evidence, the authors explained "data on sexual behavior are notoriously imprecise." Of course, many studies show some infections come from sex, but that is not at all the same as showing a majority of infections – much less almost all infections – come from sex.

Trace, test, sequence

In the years after WHO's and UNAIDS' 2004 defense of the view that sex explains almost all HIV in Africa, a lot of new and unsupportive evidence has come from studies that traced and tested sexual partners. At least three different study designs contribute useful evidence.

Sequencing HIV from a community

One of the best ways to see how much sex contributes to Africa's epidemics is to collect blood samples from a large percentage of HIV-positive people in a community, sequence collected HIV (determine the order of each HIV's constituent parts), and then look for similarities among sequences. If HIV sequences from two people are similar, one infected the other directly or indirectly through one or more other people. If people with similar sequences are or have been sexual partners, that is evidence one infected the other through sex.

Three recent studies sequenced HIV collected from large percentages of HIV-positive people in study communities in Africa, identified clusters (pairs or larger groups) of sequences that were similar, and compared clusters with information about sexual partnerships. What they found does not at all fit the view that sex explains almost all HIV infections in adults.

Specifically, the three studies identified sexual partnerships that could explain only 1.8% to 6.6% of the HIV infections they sampled and sequenced from each community (Figure 6.1). All identified sexual partners with similar sequences were spouses or long-term partners living together. Studies did not ask about and identify short-term partners, Of course, some HIV infections come from short-term partners, but if sex accounted for most HIV infections in adults, such partners would have to infect many times more people than long-term partners, which is absurd.

Figure 6.1: What do similar HIV sequences say about how many HIV infections come from sex?

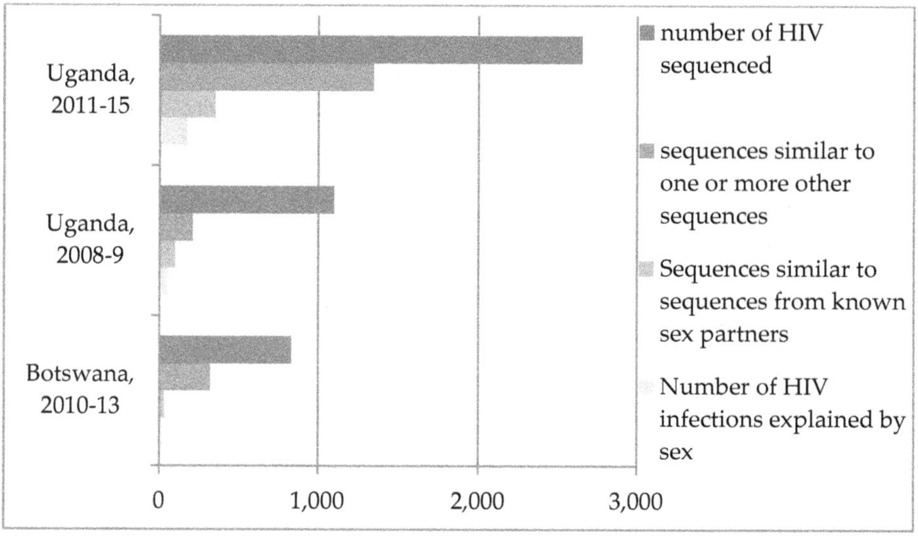

Sources: Botswana[9]; Uganda 2008-9[10]; Uganda 2011-15.[11]

One of the three studies looked at HIV collected from a community in Botswana, and two examined HIV from communities in Uganda. Here are some details.

The study in Botswana (Figure 6.1) sequenced HIV samples collected in 2010-13 from 833 adults in northeast Mochudi, a town about 50 kilometers north of Gaborone, the capital. These HIV samples represent almost half of all HIV-positive adults aged 16-64 years in the community.[9,12] Among the 833 HIV sequences, 511 were not similar to any other sequence from the community, whereas 322 were similar to one or more other sequences. In other words, 322 HIV infections were linked directly or indirectly (through other infections) to one or more infections in the community.

Thirty of these 322 sequences were in 15 pairs linking a man and a woman in a household. The study does not say if these household pairs were from spouses, but I assume so. Assuming the 15 pairs linked spouses, the study identified a sexual explanation for 15 infections – one spouse likely infected the other – but says nothing about how the first spouse got HIV. In other words, the study identified a sexual source for 1.8% (= 15/833) of HIV samples collected and sequenced. Aside from these 15 pairs, the study reports no sexual partnerships to explain why 292 (= 322 – 30) sequences from Mochudi were similar to other Mochudi sequences.

Two studies in Uganda (Figure 6.1) sequenced HIV samples collected from adults aged 15-49 years in Rakai District in southern Uganda. The first study sequenced HIV collected in 2008-9 from 1,099 adults, an estimated 42% of HIV-positive adults in 46 selected communities across Rakai District.[10] Among the 1,099 HIV sequences, 890 were not similar to any other sequence from the community, while 209 were similar to one or more other sequences. Fifty-one husband-wife pairs had similar sequences, providing a sexual explanation for 4.6% (= 51/1,099) of HIV infections with sequences in the study. Aside from 51 spouse pairs with 102 sequences, the study reported no sexual link for 107 (= 209 – 102) HIV infections with sequences similar to one or more other sequences.

The second study of HIV sequences from Rakai District used "deep sequencing," a more advanced technique that gives a more reliable picture of which HIV infections have direct or near-direct transmission links.[11] The study deep sequenced HIV samples collected during 2011-15 from 2,652 adults, an estimated 35% of HIV-positive adults in 40 selected communities across Rakai. Comparing sequences, the study assigned 1,334 sequences into clusters with one or more similar sequences. These clusters included 176 pairs linking couples. This provides a sexual explanation for 6.6% (= 176/2,652) of HIV infections with sampled sequences. There were no known sexual links to explain any of the other HIV sequence clusters.

Moreover, two of the three studies – the two from Rakai – reported percentages of married couples with similar or dissimilar HIV sequences. In both studies, when husbands and wives were both HIV-positive and their HIV was sequenced, only about half of such couples had similar HIV and therefore linked infections.[10,11] The study with deep sequencing reported the highest percentage: 53% of couples with HIV sequences from both partners had similar HIV. In other words, almost half of such couples had dissimilar HIV, showing that husbands and wives had gotten their HIV infections from different sex or blood risks.

Following people to see who gets HIV

Beginning in 1987, dozens of studies tested various ways to protect adults in Africans from HIV infections, for example, warning them about sexual risks or treating other sexual infections. These studies followed HIV-negative men and women, meeting them at intervals to see who had gotten a new HIV infection and to ask about risks.

As reported through August 2011, 44 such studies followed more than 120,000 adults for an average of almost two years each and saw more than 4,000 new HIV infections. They traced only 9.8% (393) of more than 4,000 new infections to HIV-positive sex partners.[13] To confirm new infections came from sex partners, some studies sequenced HIV from both partners. After sequencing, studies found similar HIV in sex partners for only 4.6% (186) of more than 4,000 new infections recognized in the 44 studies.

Tracing and testing contacts

For diseases such as tuberculosis and syphilis, tracing and testing is a time-honored strategy for public health agencies to find and treat new cases and to protect people who are not infected. In recent years, the strategy has been applied to HIV in Africa.

In the eight countries with the worst HIV epidemics – with more than 10% of adults infected – HIV testing programs during 2016-18 traced and tested more than 400,000 adult contacts of people who tested HIV-positive (mostly sex partners, but also needle-sharing contacts).[14] In five of these eight countries, the percentages of contacts found to be HIV-positive was less than the estimated percentages of all adults in the country who were HIV-positive in 2019 (Figure 6.2). Such results do not support the myth that almost all infected adults got HIV through sex.

Figure 6.2: Percentages of traced adult contacts testing HIV-positive vs. percentages HIV positive among all adults in the country

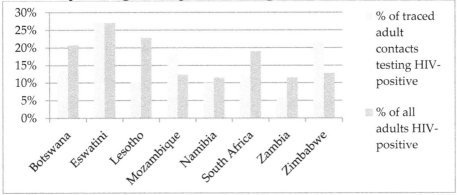

Sources: Percentages of adult contacts testing HIV-positive in 2016-18 are from CDC.[14] Percentages of all adults HIV-positive in 2019 are from UNAIDS.[15]

Sexual risks cannot explain so many new infections in young women

Another way to assess the contribution of sex to Africa's HIV epidemics is to look at groups getting a lot of new infections for which there is good information about sexual risks. In six of the eight countries in Southern Africa with the worst HIV epidemics, national surveys during 2016-17 reported women aged 15-24 years getting HIV from all causes at rates ranging from 0.46% to 1.67% per year (Figure 6.3). For those countries and years, there is sufficient information about sexual risks to estimate how much HIV they got from sex.

In South Africa, for example, in a 2016 national survey, 33% of young women aged 15-24 years said they had sex at least once in the last four weeks.[25] Although the specific women who are sexually active changes from month-to-month, considering all young women together and all months, the sexual risks that go with this behavior would be similar to 33% of all young women having sex regularly (column A Table 6.1).

What percentage of their partners were risks to transmit? First, consider partners' ages. In repeat national surveys during 2002-12, 31%-40% of sexually active women aged 15-24 years reported a recent partner at least five years older than themselves.[28] To make things simple, and to err on the high side, I assume all partners were aged 25-29 years. Second, the same 2017 South African national survey that reported new infections in women reported 12.4% of men aged 25-29 years were HIV-positive, of which 58.5% were not virally suppressed (had at least 1,000 HIV per milliliter of blood, or at least 50 HIV per drop) and were therefore a threat to transmit sexually (columns B and C in Table 6.1).[19]

For women with regular sexual exposure to HIV, how many got HIV in a year? From five studies in Africa that followed couples in which most or many wives did not know their husbands were infected, wives at risk got HIV at the rate of 11.1% per year (see Table A2.1).

Table 6.1: Estimated rates (% per year) at which women aged 15-24 years got HIV from sex, six countries in southern Africa, 2015-17

Country	% of women reporting sex last 4 weeks	% of men aged 25-29 years HIV-positive	% of such men not virally suppressed	Estimated rate women got HIV from sex (%/year)
	A	B	C	D = AxBxCx11.1%
eSwatini	27%	13.3%	51.8%	0.21%
Lesotho	24%	12.9%	56.4%	0.19%
Namibia	25%	4.2%	52.4%	0.06%
South Africa	33%	12.4%	58.5%*	0.27%
Zambia	35%	5.6%	63.2%	0.14%
Zimbabwe	34%	6.6%	73.8%	0.18%

*Percentage for men aged 25-34 years.
Sources for percentages reporting sex last four weeks by country are: eSwatini 2006-7[22]; Lesotho 2014[23]; Namibia 2013[24]; South Africa 2016[25]; Zambia 2018[26]; Zimbabwe 2015.[27] Sources for percentages of men HIV-positive and with unsuppressed viral loads by country are: eSwatini 2016-17[16]; Lesotho 2016-17[17]; Namibia 2017[18]; South Africa 2017[19]; Zambia 2016[20]; Zimbabwe 2015-16.[21]

From these data and estimates, an estimated 0.27% (= 33% x 12.4% x 58.5% x 11.1%) of young women in South Africa got HIV from sex in 2017 (column D in Table 6.1). Table 6.1 provides similar data and calculations for all six countries.

Figure 6.3 compares the estimated rates women got HIV from sex during 2015-17 (from Table 6.1) to the rates they got HIV from all risks as observed and reported by national surveys during the same years. In South Africa, for example, the estimated rate women got HIV from sex (0.27% per year) was much less than the observed 1.51% per year rate they got HV from all risks. Across all six countries, the estimated rates women got HIV from sex were much less than the observed rates at which they were getting HIV from all risks.

Figure 6.3: Comparing the estimated rates women aged 15-24 years got HIV from sex vs. the observed rates they got HIV from all risks, 2015-17

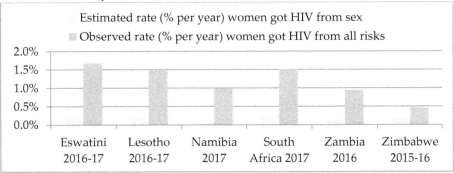

Sources: Estimated rates women got HIV from sex are from Table 6.1. Sources for rates of new infections by country are: eSwatini[16]; Lesotho[17]; Namibia[18]; South Africa[19]; Zambia[20]; Zimbabwe.[21]

If most HIV infections in young women did, indeed, come from sex, one or more of the component estimates I have used to estimate women's infections from sex must be far too low. But these estimates may also be too high. For example, I ignored condom use. Among young women who reported at least one sex partner in the previous year, from 44% to 59% said they used a condom at last sex (data from the same sources used in Table 6.1[22-27]). Did women under-report their sexual activity? Considering that more than half of young women were aged 15-19 years, there is not a lot of room for the percentages of women having sex regularly to be much greater than reported in Table 6.1.

Slow transmission through sex

Slow HIV transmission through heterosexual sex can be seen in several types of evidence from sub-Saharan Africa as well as from non-African countries.

Evidence from national surveys

In countries where low percentages of adults are HIV-positive, a husband or wife with an HIV-positive spouse has little risk to get HIV from any other source. In such countries, how fast does an HIV-positive spouse infect his or her partner? Before 2010 (before antiretroviral treatment was sufficiently common to make a big difference in sexual transmission within couples) seven national surveys in mainland sub-Saharan Africa found not more than 1.5% of adults HIV-positive. In these seven surveys, among couples in which at least one spouse was infected, the percentages of couples with both spouses infected (that is: one likely infected the other) ranged from 10% in Benin in 2006 to 19% in Guinea in 2005 (Figure 6.4).

For example, in DRC in 2007, the husband only was infected in 0.6% of couples, the wife only in 1.1% of couples, and both in 0.2% of couples. Assuming one infected the other, initially HIV-positive husbands and wives infected only 11% (= 0.2/[0.6 + 1.1 + 0.2]) of their initially HIV-negative partners.[30]

Figure 6.4: Slow HIV transmission between couples in seven African countries

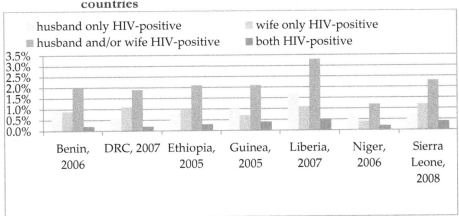

Abbreviations: DRC: Democratic Republic of the Congo.
Sources: Benin,[29] DRC,[30] Ethiopia,[31] Guinea,[32] Liberia,[33] Niger,[34] Sierra Leone.[35]

These data do not show who brought HIV into the home or how long couples lived together before one infected the other. However, we can conclude from these data that only about 15% of men and women who brought HIV into the home infected their partners (15% is the unweighted average from seven studies of the percentage of couples with both partners infected divided by the percentage with at least one infected).

If couples were living together on average for even three years after one was infected, the rate of transmission from the initially HIV-positive partners to infect 15% of their spouses would be less than 6% per year. (Even if one makes the absurd assumption that all transmission came from wives, or that all came from husbands, the rate of transmission in both cases would be less than 10% per year to reach observed percentages of both couples infected within three years.)

Couples unaware of their infections or risks

Combining results from five studies in Africa during 1989-98 in which many or most spouses did not know they were infected or at risk, initially HIV-negative men and women with HIV-positive spouses got HIV at an average rate of almost 10% per year (see Table A2.1). Some new infections that contributed to that rate may have come from sources other than HIV-positive spouses. Later studies that sequenced HIV in Rakai, Uganda, found that when both spouses were infected, HIV sequences from about half of such couples were dissimilar – husbands and wives had gotten HIV from different sources.[10,11]

Too slow!

If HIV-positive adults live 10 years without treatment, infecting sex partners at the rate of 10% per year, that could maintain a steady number of infections over time. But that would require all HIV-positive adults to be sexually active all the time with HIV-negative partners, which is not what one sees from national surveys. Many adults who are HIV-positive have HIV-positive spouses, and many others report no sex partner in the previous year. In other words, someone who is HIV-positive will on average die before he or she infects anyone through heterosexual sex.

Hence, HIV transmission through heterosexual sex is too slow to even maintain steady numbers of HIV infections in a community, much less drive an expanding epidemic. Fortunately, antiretroviral treatment (ART) extends lives. At the same time, ART reduces the risk someone with HIV will transmit through sex. With or without ART there is no heterosexual epidemic.

Similarly slow HIV transmission through heterosexual sex has been observed and reported outside Africa in countries with good information about sources of infections. In Latvia, for example, "it is difficult to observe a sustained heterosexual epidemic without continued input from an 'outside' reservoir."[36] A study in Switzerland estimated that HIV-positive heterosexuals infected an average of only 0.44 persons though sex in their lifetime, "far below the epidemic threshold."[37] In layman's terms: HIV transmission through heterosexual sex was too slow to even maintain the same number of infections over time.

Not much more HIV in sexually more active adults

In seven of the eight countries with the worst epidemics (comparable data are not available for Botswana), 6.2%-15.6% of adults aged 15-49 years reported more than one sex partner in the previous year (light grey bars in Figure 6.5). The average across the seven countries was less than 10%.

Figure 6.5: HIV infections do not concentrate in sexually more active adults

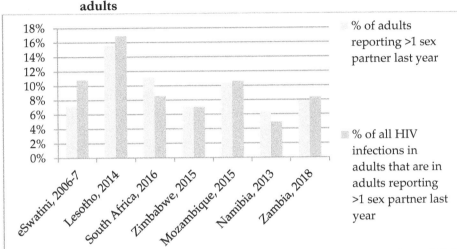

Sources: eSwatini 2006-7[22]; Lesotho 2014[23]; South Africa 2016[25]; Zimbabwe 2015[27]; Mozambique 2015[38]; Namibia 2013[24]; Zambia 2018.[26]

These sexually more active adults did not have a lot more HIV than other adults. The percentages of all HIV infections in adults that were in those who reported more than one sex partner last year (dark grey bars in Table 6.5) were similar to the percentages of adults reporting more than one partner. In Namibia and South Africa, the percentages of HIV in sexually more active adults were less than their percentage of all adults: they were less likely to be HIV-positive! And in Zimbabwe, they were equally likely to be HIV-positive.

If sex accounts for most HIV infections, HIV should concentrate in those who are more sexually active, as one sees with common sexually transmitted disease such as syphilis. But that is not what happens. Furthermore, considering the low percentages of adults reporting more than one sex partner per year, a lot of people getting HIV from sex will be staying with the partner who infected them, so their HIV has no chance to get to anyone else through sex.

What do models show?

Some proponents of the view that almost all HIV infections among adults in Africa come from sex have proposed models to show how that could be so. But to generate anything that looks like Africa's epidemics, model-builders have to assume sexual behaviors and/or rates of HIV transmission though sex that do not agree with evidence.[39] For example, when a team of experts tried to model Zambia's HIV epidemic using sexual behavior data from a national survey and the rate of HIV transmission per sex act from a study in Africa, they failed: "no epidemic could be generated."[40] To get the result they wanted they made up what they needed: "After exploring a wide range of parameters [sexual behaviors and transmission per sex act], we found a combination giving a good fit to the age and sex patterns of prevalence in 2001." To make their model generate something that looked like Zambia's epidemic, they assumed men had more commercial sex than they reported and a higher than observed rate of HIV transmission per sex act. But what did that prove? Adjusting assumptions to reach desired conclusions can "prove" almost anything: cows fly, pigs lay eggs, all HIV in adults comes from heterosexual sex, etc.

Why has the myth lasted so long?

In countries where a lot of adults are HIV-positive, HIV prevention programs should warn people to avoid HIV from sex. But to make that point stick, such programs do not have to say all HIV comes from sex. Similarly, clergy, parents, and others who want to discourage pre-marital or extra-marital sex may cite HIV as a danger for those who "misbehave." But to discourage sex outside marriage, clergy and parents do not have to say all HIV comes from sex, just that some comes from sex.

So why has the myth lasted so long? Health professionals appear to be the only group delivering HIV prevention messages that has any reason to promote the myth. Blaming sex distracts attention from unexplained infections and bloodborne risks. That allows health aid agencies and governments to extend healthcare programs – immunizations, antenatal care, hospital deliveries – without having to take the effort to make health care reliably safe and without having to be accountable to patients.

The myth that almost all HIV-infections among adults in Africa comes from sex emerged in the face of contradictory evidence and continues despite more such evidence. John Potterat, a veteran of years of debates in medical journals about HIV from sex and bloodborne risks in the US and Africa has written a short, detailed criticism of bad science defending the myth.[41]

References

[1] Pinching A. AIDS and Africa: lessons for us all. *J Roy Soc Med* 1986; 79: 501-503.

[2] Hrdy DB. Cultural practices contributing to the transmission of human immunodeficiency virus in Africa. *Rev Infect Dis* 1987; 9: 1109-1119.

[3] Piot P, Plummer FA, Mhalue FS, et.al. AIDS: an international perspective. *Science* 1988; 239: 573-579.

[4] Chin J, Sato PA, Mann JM. Projections of HIV infections and AIDS cases to the year 2000. *Bull World Health Org* 1990;68:1–11.

[5] Gisselquist D, Potterat JJ, Brody S, Vachon F. Let it be sexual: how health care transmission of AIDS in Africa was ignored. *Int J STD AIDS* 2003; 14: 148-161.

[6] Wellings K, Collumbien M, Slaymaker E, et al. Sexual behaviour in context: a global perspective. *Lancet* 2006; 368: 1706-1728.

[7] Schmid GP, Buve A, Mugyenyi P, et al. Transmission of HIV-infection in sub-Saharan Africa and effect of elimination of unsafe injections. *Lancet* 2004; 363: 482-488.

[8] Gisselquist D, Potterat JJ, Heterosexual transmission of HIV in Africa: an empiric estimate. *Int J STD AIDS* 2003; 14: 162-173.

[9] Novitsky V, Bussmann H, Okui L, et al. Estimated age and gender profile of individuals missed by a home-based HIV testing and counseling campaign in a Botswana community. *J Int AIDS Soc* 2015; 18: 19918.

[10] Grabowski MK, Lessler J, Redd AD, et al. The role of viral introductions in sustaining community-based HIV epidemics in rural Uganda: evidence from spatial clustering, phylogenetics, and egocentric transmission models. *PLoS* 2014; 11: e1001610.

[11] Ratmann O, Grabowski MK, Hall M, et al. Inferring HIV-1 transmission networks and sources of epidemic spread in Africa with deep-sequence phylogenetic analysis. *Nat Commun* 2019; 10: 1411.

[12] Novitsky V, Kuhnert K, Moyo S, et al. Phylodynamic analysis of HIV sub-epidemics in Mochudi, Botswana. *Epidemics* 2015; 13: 44-55.

[13] Gisselquist D. Randomized controlled trials for HIV/AIDS prevention among men and women in Africa: untraced infections, unasked questions, and unreported data. *Social Science Research Network* [internet] 9 October 2011. Available at: https://papers.ssrn.com/sol3/papers.cfm?abstract_id=1940999 (accessed 9 June 2020).

[14] Lasry A, Medley A, Behel S, et al. Scaling up testing for human immunodeficiency virus infection among contacts of index patients -- 20 Countries, 2016–2018. *MMWR Morb Mort Wkly Rep* 2019; 68: 474-477.

[15] UNAIDS. HIV estimates with uncertainty bounds 1990-2019. Geneva: UNAIDS, 2020.

[16] ICAP. *Swaziland HIV incidence measurement survey 2 (SHIMS2) 2016-2017: Final Report.* New York (NY): ICAP, Columbia University, 2019.

[17] ICAP. *Lesotho population-based HIV impact assessment (LePHIA) 2016-2017: Final report.* New York (NY): ICAP, Columbia University, 2019.

[18] ICAP. *Namibia Population-based HIV Impact Assessment (NAMPHIA) 2017: Final Report.* New York (NY): ICAP, Columbia University, 2019.

[19] Simbayi LC, Zuma K, Zungu N, et al. *South African National HIV Prevalence, Incidence, Behaviour and Communications Survey 2017.* Cape Town: HSRC; 2019.

[20] ICAP. *Zambia Population-based HIV Impact Assessment (ZAMPHIA) 2016: Final Report.* New Yok (NY): ICAP, Columbia University, 2019.

[21] ICAP. *Zimbabwe Population-based HIV Impact Assessment (ZIMPHIA) 2015-2016: Final Report.* New York (NY): ICAP, Columbia University, 2019.

[22] Macro International. *Swaziland Demographic and Health Survey 2006-07.* Calverton (MD): Macro International; 2008.

[23] ICF International. *Lesotho Demographic and Health Survey 2014.* Rockville (MD): ICF; 2016.

[24] ICF International. *The Namibia demographic and health survey 2013.* Rockville (MD): ICF International, 2014.

[25] ICF. *South Africa Demographic and Health Survey 2016.* Rockville [1] (MD): ICF; 2019.

[26] ICF. *Zambia Demographic and Health Survey 2018.* Rockville (MD): ICF, 2019.

[27] ICF International. *Zimbabwe Demographic and Health Survey 2015: Final Report.* Rockville (MD): ICF International, 2016.

[28] Evans M, Risher K, Zungu N, et al. Age-disparate sex and HIV risk for young women from 2002 to 2012 in South Africa. *J Int AIDS Soc* 2016; 19: 21310.

[29] Macro International. *Enquête Démographique et de Santé (EDSB-III) - Bénin 2006.* Calverton, (MD): Macro International. 2007

30 Macro International. *Enquête Démographique et de Santé, République Démocratique du Congo 2007*. Calverton (MD): Macro International, 2008.

31 OCR Macro. *Ethiopia Demographic and Health Survey 2005*. Calverton (MD): OCR Macro, 2006.

32 ORC Macro. *Enquête Démographique et de Santé, Guinée 2005*. Calverton (MD): ORC Macro, 2006

33 Macro International. *Liberia Demographic and Health Survey 2007*. Calverton (MD): Macro International, 2008.

34 Macro International. *Enquête Démographique et de Santé at a Indicateurs Multiples du Niger 2006*. Calverton (MD): Macro International, 2007.

35 ICF Macro. *Sierra Leone Demographic and Health Survey 2008*. Calverton (MD): ICF Macro, 2009.

36 Graw F, Leitner T, Ribeiro RM. Agent-based and phylogenetic analyses reveal how HIV-1 moves between risk groups: injecting drug users sustain the heterosexual epidemic in Latvia. *Epidemics* 2012; 4: 104-116.

37 Turk T, Bachmann N, Kadelka C, et al. Assessing the danger of self-sustained HIV epidemics in heterosexuals by population based phylogenetic cluster analysis. *eLife* [internet] 2017; 6: e28721.

38 ICF. *Inquérito de Indicadores de Imunização, Malária e HIV/SIDA em Moçambique 2015*. Rockville (MD); ICF, 2018.

39 Deuchert E, Brody S. Plausible and implausible parameters for mathematical modeling of nominal heterosexual HIV transmission. *Ann Epidemiol* 2007; 17: 237-244.

40 Leclerc PM, Matthews AP, Garenne ML. Fitting the HIV epidemic in Zambia: a two-sex micro-simulation model. *PLoS One 2009*; 4: e5439.

41 Potterat JJ. Why Africa? the puzzle of intense HIV transmission in heterosexuals. In: Potterat JJ. *Seeking the positives: a life spent on the cutting edge of public health*. North Charleston (SC): Createspace, 2015. pp 175-229.

CHAPTER SEVEN

Errors and Delays in Responses to Africa's HIV Epidemics

After decades of errors and delays in responses to Africa's HIV epidemics, new policies and programs extending testing, antiretroviral treatment (ART), and prevention of mother-to-child transmission are saving lives. AIDS deaths per year among adults and children in sub-Saharan Africa reached an estimated peak of 1.31 million in 2004, but have since fallen 66% to 440,000 in 2019.[1]

New infections per year have fallen as well, but not as much. Estimated new infections peaked in 1996-97 at 1.97 million, then fell 51% to 970,000 in 2019. An old and ongoing error – seeing unexplained HIV infections without asking for investigations to find and stop their source – largely explains continuing high numbers of new infections.

Continuing high numbers of new infections are motivating new errors: International and foreign health organizations are promoting dangerous and unnecessary medical interventions to the African public as ways to reduce HIV from sexual risks.

Old and continuing errors in responses to Africa's HIV epidemics have been particularly harmful for women.

Early errors

Error: accepting HIV from health care

After finding HIV-positive children with HIV-negative mothers in DRC and Rwanda in 1984-86, experts from the US and Europe accepted that reuse of contaminated instruments in health care would continue to infect an unknown number of Africans with HIV (Chapter 3). This was decided without investigations, which were required to protect public health in any case, but which would have also given not only researchers and public health officials but also the general public some idea of the scale of the problem.

Africa's epidemics might have developed differently if experts had instead recommended governments to investigate to find and fix bloodborne risks. Although governments of DRC and Rwanda may not have investigated at the time, a clear and repeated recommendation could have made it easier for one or more governments in sub-Saharan Africa to investigate in later months and years. In addition, experts could have challenged donors to immediately stop accepting unsafe skin-piercing procedures in health aid programs. That did not happen. Unsafe immunizations injections continued on a massive scale until the end of the century (Chapter 3). There was no urgency to change.

With an alternate response, experts could have (and should have) articulated the hypothesis that HIV transmission through skin-piercing medical and cosmetic procedures could be driving Africa's HIV epidemics. (A hypothesis does not say anything is true, but rather that it might be.) That hypothesis agreed with evidence available at the time from the US and other countries outside sub-Saharan Africa with good information about sources of HIV infections. In the US, for example, as of 1988, 62% of AIDS cases were in men who have sex with men (MSM; excluding MSM who were also injection drug users [IDUs]); 31% were in people with blood exposures (IDUs, people who had received blood transfusions or blood products, and people with other healthcare risks), and only 2.8% were attributed to heterosexual contact, mostly in women partnered with IDUs and MSM. (These percentages exclude small numbers of HIV-positive people from Haiti and Africa whose risks were not known.)[2]

From the perspective of 2020, the hypothesis that bloodborne risks drive Africa's epidemics fits accumulating evidence (Chapter 6). If in the mid-1980s experts had respected that hypothesis and had encouraged governments to investigate unexplained infections, the reduction of HIV transmission through skin-piercing medical procedures might have changed the course of Africa's HIV epidemics. Africa's epidemics might well have developed just like HIV epidemics in the US and elsewhere: more HIV-positive men than women, and far less than 1% of adults infected. Considering that the risks accounting for most HIV infections outside Africa (MSM and IDU) are not so evident in Africa, the percentage of adults who are HIV-positive in Africa should be lower than elsewhere. But that is not what happened.

Error: blaming HIV-positive Africans for sexual misbehavior

Beginning in the 1980s, HIV prevention messages for Africans focused on sex. The claim that almost all HIV infections came from sex had a paralyzing effect on HIV prevention in Africa. Based on their sexual behaviors, most people considered themselves to be safe (see Annex 1). People did not realize they were at risk to get HIV from skin-piercing procedures in hospitals and clinics. And so HIV spread, unrecognized, through the general population. Paradoxically, focusing on sex increased sexual risks; warnings about bloodborne risks as well as sex would have alerted people that virgins or monogamous spouses might be infected, so that sex with anyone could be a risk for HIV.

Public health messages blaming almost all HIV infections on sex encouraged people to consider an HIV infection to be a sign of sexual behaviors – pre-marital or extra-marital sex, buying or selling sex – widely considered to be misbehaviors in societies with conservative social norms. Such messages extended into Africa stigmatizing opinions that were common in the US and Europe: that HIV infections came from "bad" behaviors.

WOMANKIND Worldwide defines sexual bullying to include: "a range of behaviours such as… spreading rumours about someone's sexuality or sexual experiences they have had or not had…"[3] Public health messages that blamed almost all HIV infections on sex, despite evidence to the contrary, were equivalent to malicious and unfounded rumors. Although such public messages were impersonal, they encouraged people to think they knew something about the sexual behavior of specific HIV-positive people and to believe and spread similarly unfounded rumors about them.

Error: discouraging HIV tests

As the AIDS epidemic emerged in the US in the 1980s, many MSM wanted to keep their male-male sexual behavior secret. Their desire for secrecy led to "AIDS exceptionalism." HIV tests were considered sensitive and dangerous, because an HIV-positive result could expose a man as an MSM. Public health officials treated test results as personal secrets, recorded and reported without names. Tracing and testing sex partners, which was standard for syphilis and other sexually transmitted disease, was seldom done for HIV infections.

Accepting and extending AIDS exceptionalism into Africa, WHO's Global Programme on AIDS cautioned that "National AIDS programmes that decide to develop voluntary testing and counselling services where none now exist should proceed cautiously by initiating a trial project."[4] When a 1994 article in *The Lancet* proposed "voluntary home testing" to allow people in developing countries to see if they or their sexual partners were infected,[5] experts from WHO's Global Programme on AIDS attacked. They characterized testing as the "The policeman's response to HIV/AIDS" and rejected the suggestion that testing could help to slow HIV transmission as an "old fallacy."[6] But the only article they cited to support that statement reported "substantial risk reduction among heterosexual partners with one infected partner."[7]

AIDS exceptionalism influenced international and foreign organizations to recommend special arrangements for HIV tests, including counseling before and after. Because of all the regulatory obstacles together with limited donor support, testing facilities were few and far between, and getting an HIV test was difficult in most African countries until some years after 2000. Because public health messages blamed HIV on sexual risks that most Africans did not have, most people saw no reason to go through the trouble of getting a test.

Not testing and tracing partners of persons found HIV-positive was a limited problem in the US and other rich countries where infections concentrated in populations with specific behaviors (MSM and IDU). But in Africa, limited testing left many millions of people in the general population unaware of their infections (Figure 7.1) and not knowing if their partners were infected. As late as 2000, Peter Piot, the head of UNAIDS at the time, estimated only about 5% of HIV-positive Africans knew they were infected.[8]

Error: not preventing mother-to-child transmission

If a woman who is not aware she is HIV-positive has a baby and breastfeeds it for 1-2 years, there is roughly a 35% chance she will transmit HIV to her baby, 20% at birth and 15% from breastfeeding. Almost all of that can be prevented. As early as 1994, a study found that giving women the antiretroviral drug zidovudine (AZT or ZVD) as pills for five months when pregnant and intravenously during delivery, and then giving the baby ZDV could reduce by two-thirds mother-to-child HIV transmission at birth. This was widely adopted almost immediately in rich countries. In the US, for example, more than 60% of HIV-positive pregnant women received ZDV in 1996.[14]

Figure 7.1: Percentages of HIV-positive people in sub-Saharan Africa knowing they are infected, getting ART, and getting PMTCT

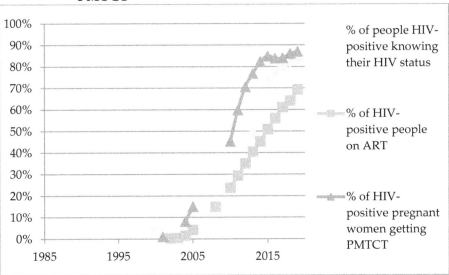

Abbreviations: ART: antiretroviral treatment; PMTCT: prevention of mother-to-child transmission.
Sources: Percentages of people knowing they are infected in 2015-19, pregnant women getting PMTCT, and adults on ART in 2010-19 are from UNAIDS[1]. Other sources for percentages knowing they are infected are: 2000 from Piot[8] and 2013 from UNAIDS.[9] Other sources for HIV-positive people on ART are: 2002-5 from UNAIDS[10] and 2008 from WHO et al.[11] Other sources for pregnant women getting PMTCT are: 2001 from WHO,[12] 2004 from Partnership for Maternal, Newborn & Child health,[13] and 2005 from WHO et al.[11]

Giving HIV-positive women intravenous ZDV during delivery to protect their babies was considered too difficult for Africa. In any case, much better – and easier – drug plans soon followed. Two trials in 1998 showed that a shorter course of oral ZDV or single oral doses of nevirapine, another antiretroviral, to mother and baby reduced mother-to-child transmission by about 50%. Combined, they gave better results. Regimens of three oral drugs to the mother and ZDV and/or nevirapine to the baby did even better, cutting transmission at birth to near 1% as early as 2004 in Thailand.[15]

In 1998, USAID proposed to scale up programs to prevent mother-to-child HIV transmission (PMTCT) in Africa. In 1999, interested donors established an Inter-Agency Task Team on PMTCT. In 2000, WHO recommended giving HIV-positive pregnant women and babies antiretroviral drugs to protect babies. But several more years went by before more than a small minority of HIV-positive pregnant women in Africa could get the drugs needed to protect their babies (Figure 7.1).

Error: not allowing antiretroviral treatment (ART) for Africans

Giving HIV-positive people antiretroviral drugs to suppress their infections began on a big scale in the US in 1996. From 1995 to 1998, deaths from AIDS in the US fell by 64%.[16] In 2003, seven years after antiretroviral treatment (ART) had been widely adopted in rich countries, less than 1% of HIV-positive Africans were on ART (Figure 7.1). The delay in getting drugs to Africans was due to artificial barriers: intellectual property rights forced market prices far above production costs; and national regulations controlled imports. At the end of the 1990s and early 2000's, the usual price for a year's supply of ART drugs for one person was $10,000-$15,000 in rich countries. These prices far exceeded the cost to produce the drugs.

Early errors violate human rights

Not finding and fixing bloodborne risks in health care and not warning Africans about such risks violates human rights (Chapter 3). Blaming HIV-positive Africans for sexual misbehavior violates human rights.

In 1994, Jonathan Mann, an influential architect of these errors, assessed that lack of respect for human rights contributed to HIV epidemics: "the evolving HIV/AIDS pandemic has shown a consistent pattern through which discrimination, marginalization, stigmatization and, more generally, a lack of respect for the human rights and dignity of individuals and groups heightens their vulnerability to becoming exposed to HIV."[17] Although Mann did not intend it, his criticism applies to the double standard in healthcare safety and victim blaming (and stigmatizing) he had helped to introduce into responses to Africa's HIV epidemics. Aside from those human rights violations, his assessment did not fit sub-Saharan Africa, where HIV invaded the general population, and where infections were more common in people with more than average wealth and education.

2000-05: Turning some corners, correcting some errors

Testing, preventing mother-to-child transmission, and treatment (ART) arrived after long delays due to policies and regulations blocking private initiatives as well as to donors and governments taking time to design and fund public programs.

Finally allowing and promoting testing!

In 2002, Kevin De Cock and colleagues published an impassioned criticism of AIDS exceptionalism in Africa: the current response to Africa's HIV epidemics was not adequate for a "public health and infectious disease emergency" which was the leading cause of death in Africa. As part of an adequate response, "routine diagnostic HIV testing will have to become standard practice in medical care."[18] In the ensuing debate about whether and how to increase HIV testing, De Cock's and colleagues' proposal was characterized as "provider initiated testing" or "opt out" testing – with doctors routinely testing patients for HIV as they would for other conditions, and with patients opting out if they wished.

    Most African governments readily accepted provider initiated testing. During 2003-8, 37 African countries established policies for provider initiated testing in at least some settings.[19] By 2010, almost all African countries had adopted provider initiated testing for pregnant women, and more than half had done so for all adults attending a health facility. On the other hand, WHO and UNAIDS had more trouble letting go of AIDS exceptionalism. In 2004 and 2007 they endorsed provider initiated testing in some settings (for example, in antenatal care) but with caveats, including detailed pre-test counselling[20] and the availability of a "recommended package of HIV prevention, treatment and care."[21]

Whatever the caveats, the battle was won. AIDS exceptionalism was defeated in Africa. Expanding programs to prevent mother-to-child transmission and to keep HIV-positive Africans alive with ART soon ended opposition to provider initiated testing. The percentage of HIV-positive Africans aware of their infections reached an estimated 49% in 2013 and 83% in 2019.

Aside from signaling a need for treatment, testing has an important role to play in preventing sexual transmission. This role was overlooked in Africa for decades. Not until 2012 did WHO finally endorse couple counseling: "Couples and partners should be offered voluntary HIV testing and counselling with support for mutual disclosure."[22] Four years later, in 2016, WHO made further recommendations to give testing an even bigger role in HIV prevention. Specifically, WHO urged governments: to help people who test HIV-positive tell their sex partners; and to allow sales of self-testing kits.[23] In 2016, the US CDC initiated programs with partner organizations throughout Africa to trace and test contacts of people who tested HIV-positive.[24]

Self-testing can make a big difference. In a 2017-18 study in South Africa, young women given self-testing kits (for own use, with extras to distribute) were much more likely to test and to get their sex partners and others to test compared to young women referred for tests at government clinics.[25] One continuing snag with respect to testing has been the myth that almost all infections come from sex. Even with an estimated 83% of people who are HIV-positive in sub-Saharan Africa knowing their status as of 2019 (Figure 7.1), that still leaves one-sixth who are not aware. Many do not think to test because they have had no or low sexual risks.

Prevention of mother-to-child transmission (PMTCT)

At the beginning of the twenty-first century, the Irish singer Bono got together with Jesse Helms, a notoriously conservative US Senator, to promote prevention of mother-to-child transmission (PMTCT) in Africa. In 2002, the US government approved $500 million for PMTCT. One year later, President Bush proposed $15 billion over five years for HIV/AIDS programs in 15 countries (12 in Africa). Congress agreed.

The $15 billion went through a new office, the Presidents' Emergency Program for AIDS Relief (PEPFAR). Along with other activities, PEPFAR supported PMTCT.

Through 2005, many mothers and babies received single doses of nevirapine. As PMTCT programs expanded, drug regimens got better, further cutting HIV transmission from mothers to babies. WHO's 2004, 2006, and 2010 recommendations for PMTCT proposed various options for drugs to give mothers and babies.[26,27] In 2012, WHO recommended starting all HIV-positive pregnant women on ART, to be continued for life. WHO called this the B+ option.[28] ART for life can reduce a mother's risks to infect her baby at birth and through breastfeeding to only a few percent.

PMTCT has made a huge difference in Africa, but it was delayed. In 2010, 12 years after research had confirmed that several simple oral regimens protected babies, less than half of HIV-positive pregnant women in sub-Saharan Africa received drugs for PMTCT. In those 12 years, more than four million children aged 0-14 years in Africa got HIV (UNAIDS estimates). The extension of PMTCT reduced the estimated annual number of new infections in children age 0-14 years by over 60%, from 430,000 in 2000 to 126,000 in 2019 (Figure 7.2; UNAIDS estimates). Considering what can be achieved with B+ (putting pregnant women on ART for life), numbers of new infections in children can go much lower.

Figure 7.2: More testing, ART, and PMTCT reduce AIDS deaths and new infections

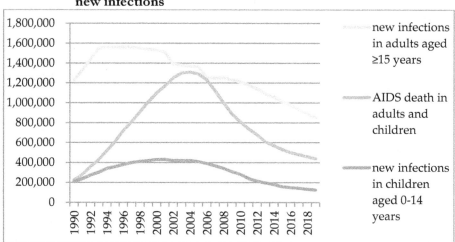

Abbreviations: ART: antiretroviral therapy. PMTCT: prevention of mother to child transmission.
Source: UNAIDS.[1]

Antiretroviral treatment (ART)

From 1996, when ART was introduced in rich countries, through 2004, more than eight million Africans died of AIDS. Because AIDS in Africa concentrates in urban and mid-level or wealthier adults and in wealthier countries, the political implications were untenable. AIDS in Africa was killing community and national leaders, their families, and friends.

Shortly after ART was adopted in rich countries, companies in Brazil, Thailand, and India began to produce generic drugs with or even without the approval of companies holding patents. Because of legal barriers created by intellectual property rights, it took time for generic antiretroviral drugs to get to Africa.

In 1998, Partners in Health, a US-based non-government organization led by Paul Farmer and Jim Kim, began to provide ART to poor Haitians, demonstrating the feasibility of getting ART to Africans.[29] In 2001, Cipla, an Indian company producing generic antiretroviral drugs, offered to sell them to African governments for $600 per patient per year and to Partners in Health for $350 per patient per year.[30]

In 2003, Jim Kim moved to WHO. He became head of WHO's AIDS office in early 2004. With Kim's lead, WHO and UNAIDS in 2003 initiated an ambitious 3 by 5 program: to provide ART to "3 million people living with HIV/AIDS in poor countries by the end of 2005."[31] In three years, from 2002 to 2005, the percentage of HIV-positive Africans taking ART increased from 0.3% to 4.2%. Although the 3 by 5 program missed its target by a few years, it transformed attitudes about ART for Africans – they were going to get ART. In pressing international agencies, companies, and donors to figure out how to get ART to Africans, Paul Farmer and Jim Kim made a huge contribution to Africans' health.

In 2003, WHO recommended ART for only a minority of HIV-positive people, those with already weak immune systems, identified by having less than 200 CD4 cells (a type of white blood cell) per cubic millimeter of blood (about 1/50th of a drop). Over the next 11 years, WHO and UNAIDS recommended ART for progressively more HIV-positive people with newer infections and stronger immune systems.

In 2014, WHO and UNAIDS recommended ART for everyone who is HIV-positive. This recommendation was motivated in large part by the recognition that people with less virus in their blood (with suppressed viral loads, commonly defined as having less than 1,000 HIV per milliliter, or about 50 HIV per drop of blood) almost never transmitted HIV to sex partners. ART for all HIV-positive adults and children has been promoted as "treatment as prevention" and described as "test and treat."

WHO and UNAIDS packaged their recommendations for ART into 90-90-90 goals for 2020: 90% of people who are HIV-positive know it; 90% who know are on ART; and 90% of people on ART have suppressed viral loads.[9] In 2016, the UN General Assembly endorsed 90-90-90 goals for 2020.[32] Although not many countries have been on track to reach these targets, they motivated rapid expansion of testing and treatment in countries with the worst epidemics. Through 2019, the percentage of HIV-positive Africans taking ART increased to an estimated 69%. Among the four countries with the worst epidemics, eSwatini (96% on ART) and Botswana (82%) did better than South Africa (70%) and Lesotho (65% on ART).[1]

With governments and donors aiming for 90-90-90 targets, large majorities of HIV-positive people are getting tested and treated, allowing near normal life expectancies and opportunities. But the continuing treatment challenges are daunting, including: reaching more people; changing ART drugs as people develop resistance and as better drugs come along; and helping people with HIV deal with drug side-effects and HIV-related health problems.

Old errors beget new ones

In contrast to good progress with treatment, prevention has lagged. In 2016, the UN General Assembly set a target to cut new HIV infections among adults aged 15 years and older in sub-Saharan Africa to 277,000 in 2020 (see para 65a in[32]). According to UNAIDS' estimates for 2019, this target will be badly missed. Estimated new infections among adults aged 15-49 years in sub-Saharan Africa fell only 30% from 1,210,000 in 2010 to 850,000 in 2019 (Figure 7.2).[1] Despite disappointing progress, there is room for optimism. Based on the evidence presented in Chapter 6, there is reason to hope that the UN's target for 2020 and even much greater cuts in numbers of new infections could be achieved within several years through large reductions in bloodborne transmission guided by investigations of unexplained infections.

Based on the same evidence from Chapter 6, the UN's proposed reductions in new infections are likely to be impossible if all the cuts have to come from sexual transmission. All along sex has very likely been responsible for a minority of HIV infections in Africa. Moreover, the risk to get HIV from sex is a personal risk that people can and do control with multiple options: testing partners, using condoms or avoiding people who may be infected, and ART as prevention for recognized HIV-positive partners. In recent years, people have gotten even more able to control their sexual risks with governments promoting couple counseling and allowing self-testing kits[25] and with more HIV-positive people taking ART.

How much sexual transmission continues to slip through all the various ways people have to protect themselves? Probably not much. Nevertheless, ongoing old errors – ignoring HIV from health care and blaming sex – have led to new errors. These new errors are dangerous and unnecessary medical interventions proposed to reduce what is already a much diminished number of sexual transmissions. The situation is akin to the old joke about someone looking for lost keys on one side of the road under the streetlight because that is where the light is rather than on the dark side of the road where he dropped them.

New error: circumcising men to reduce their risk to get HIV from sex

In 2007, WHO and UNAIDS recommended "male circumcision should be recognized as an additional, important strategy for the prevention of heterosexually acquired HIV infection in men."[33] Subsequently, WHO and UNAIDS endorsed programs to circumcise 20 million men in 14 countries in sub-Saharan Africa during 2008-15.[34] After 11.7 million circumcisions were reported through 2015, UNAIDS set a new target to circumcise another 25 million men in 15 countries during 2016-20.[35,36] Through 2017, the US government supported more than 80% of these circumcisions.[37]

WHO's and UNAIDS' recommendation was based on three studies in Africa that reported circumcised men were less likely to get HIV than intact (uncircumcised men). But what happened in those studies? In two of the studies, men who reported no sexual risks (no partners or 100% condom use) got HIV at rates more than half as fast as the rates for men who reported any unprotected sex.[38,39] The third study did not report men's sexual risks.[40] One study tested most wives, but has not said if the wives of men getting new infections during the study were known to be HIV-positive or HIV-negative.[39,41]

But criticizing these studies – how they were badly managed and reported – does not get to the heart of the problem with circumcising millions of men to prevent HIV. Insofar as sex is a risk, men already have multiple options to protect themselves. And because there is overwhelming evidence bloodborne risks – most likely in medical settings – drive Africa's epidemics (Chapter 6), it is irresponsible to put millions of men at risk for HIV and other bad outcomes from unnecessary operations.[42,43]

New error: promoting pre-exposure prophylaxis (PrEP) to women in the general population to protect them from HIV via sex

Giving HIV-negative people drugs to prevent infection is known as "pre-exposure prophylaxis" or PrEP. The most common PrEP drugs currently in use are oral, taken daily or intermittently around the time someone is exposed to HIV. Other PrEP options may be useful in the future. PrEP can protect people exposed to HIV from either sex or blood.[44,45] In 2015, WHO proposed offering PrEP to "all population groups" getting HIV at rates of at least 3% per year, or even less if prevention costs less than lifetime treatment after infection.[46]

Most PrEP users in the world are MSM. Within Africa, some programs target PrEP to MSM and sex workers, who have sexual risks not common in the general population. Those programs are as sensible in Africa as elsewhere.

However, much of the effort to promote PrEP in Africa is based on the expectation that widespread PrEP use could protect women in the general population, especially young women, from getting HIV via sex and thereby have a big impact on numbers of new HIV infections. Those hopes are ill-founded. According to the best available evidence (Chapter 6), most women's infections likely come from bloodborne risks; and women already have multiple options to protect themselves from HIV via sex.

In recent studies, efforts to persuade women in the general population in Africa to use PrEP to protect themselves from sexual risks have been running into a wall of indifference. For example, during 2009-12, two trials among women in Kenya, South Africa, Tanzania, Uganda, and Zimbabwe recruited HIV-negative women, gave some women PrEP and others a placebo (a pill designed to do nothing), and then followed and retested them to see if PrEP protected them from HIV. The trials failed: women got HIV at similar high rates with either PrEP or the placebo.[47,48] Some women said they skipped pills when they had no sexual risks, such as when their partners were away.[49] Did women who skipped pills get HIV from bloodborne risks? Neither study considered that possibility or reported women's bloodborne risks.

Similarly, a 2017-18 study promoted PrEP to pregnant women and mothers in Kenya to protect them from HIV via sex.[50] Twenty-two percent accepted a month of pills, but less than 3% continued for six months. Clearly, most women were not interested. More than half of those who continued had partners of unknown HIV status, something that could have been resolved by testing the partners, thereby saving women from the side effects and nuisances of PrEP.

Many women did not like PrEP's common side effects (nausea, vomiting, tiredness, etc.). Reports from these studies do not say what women knew or thought about less common but more serious side effects (weaker bones, possible kidney damage).

Generalizing from studies to date, most women are not interested in PrEP to prevent HIV from sex. In some special situations, of course, some women may want PrEP to protect them during sex, for example, if they want to get pregnant by a man with an uncontrolled viral load.

Because much if not most of women's HIV infections likely come from bloodborne risks, PrEP could be considered to protect women from bloodborne risks. Any thoughts about how that might be done are beyond the scope of this book.

Not protecting women

International and foreign organizations and governments have not done what is needed to protect women, and have even harmed them:

- No government has investigated unexplained HIV infections in self-declared virgins (Chapter 4) or new HIV infections in young or pregnant women getting HIV at rates too high to be explained by sex (Chapters 4 and 6).
- Donors promote Depo-Provera injections for birth control despite evidence Depo use increases women's risk to get HIV by 40%-50% (Annex 2).
- Donors and governments promote circumcising men, even though the one study that looked at the matter found that newly circumcised HIV-positive men were 49% more likely to infect their wives than were intact men (the study recorded only 25 new infections, so that result may be a statistical accident).[51]
- Among couples in Africa in which only one partner is infected, the wife is often the one infected (Figure 6.4). The myth that almost all HIV infections come from sex threatens women with disrespect and

suspicion about their sexual behavior and truthfulness – adding insult to injury.

The consequences of such policies have been tragic. Women account for more than 60% of HIV-positive adults in Africa. In the four countries with the worst epidemics, by the time women are 20-24 years old, from 14.6% to 20.9% are infected, and by the time they are 35-39 years old, from 39.4% to 54.2% are infected (Figure 7.3). These are national averages from the latest national surveys! HIV/AIDS policies and programs have failed them and harmed them.

Figure 7.3: Percentages of young women HIV-positive and maximum percentages of women HIV-positive by 5-year age cohort*

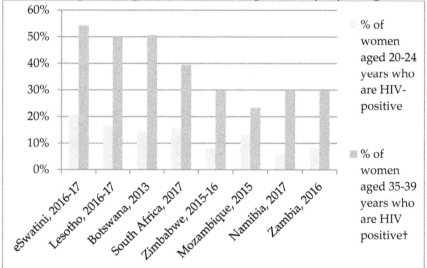

*Data from all eight countries with more than 10% of adults HIV-positive. Maximum percentages HIV-positive are for women aged 40-44 years in Zambia and Zimbabwe and 45-49 years in Namibia.
Sources: eSwatini[52]; Lesotho[53]; Botswana[54]; South Africa[55]; Zimbabwe[56]; Mozambique[57]; Namibia[58]; and Zambia.[59]

What happens next?

I end this book as I began. I hope that what I have written here will help people who are aware of unexplained HIV infections in themselves, their families, or friends to get others in their communities to believe them and to join them in digging for answers. I hope that by working together, communities aware of unexplained infections will be able to convince their governments to investigate to protect public health.

Africa has outspoken media and strong civil society organizations, including churches, political parties, universities, and business associations. When people in a community ask for help with an investigation, they may initially face opposition from parts of the government attentive to national, foreign, and international health experts and organizations. But with support from local media and civil society organizations, I expect government officials can be persuaded to do right by their citizens, to help them investigate to protect public health.

References

1 UNAIDS. HIV estimates with uncertainty bounds 1990-2019. Geneva: UNAIDS, 2020.
2 Centers for Disease Control and Prevention (CDC). *HIV/AIDS surveillance: AIDS cases reported through December 1988*. Atlanta: CDC, 1989.
3 WOMANKIND Worldwide. *Stop sexual bullying: preventing violence, promoting equality, act now*. London: WOMANKIND Worldwide, 2010.
4 Global Programme on AIDS. Statement from the consultation on HIV testing and counselling for HIV infection, Geneva 16-18 November 1992. Geneva: WHO, 1993.
5 Frerichs RR. Personal screening for HIV in developing countries. *Lancet* 1994; 343: 960-96.
6 Mertens TE, Smith GD, Van Praag E. Home testing for HIV. *Lancet* 1994; 343: 1293.
7 Higgins DL, Galavotti C, O'Reilly KR, et al. Evidence for the effects of HIV antibody testing and counseling on risk behaviors. *JAMA* 1991; 266: 2419-2429.
8 Great Britain, House of Commons, International Development Committee. *Third Report, HIV/AIDS: The impact on social and economic*

development, vol. 2 (HC 354-II). London: House of Commons, 2001. Evidence of Peter Piot on 18 July 2000.

[9] UNAIDS. *90-90-90: an ambitious treatment target to help end the AIDS epidemics.* Geneva: UNAIDS, 2014.

[10] UNAIDS. *Report on the Global AIDS epidemic.* Geneva: UNAIDS, 2006.

[11] WHO, UNAIDS, UNICEF. *Towards universal access: scaling up priority HIV/AIDS interventions in the health sector: progress report 2010.* Geneva: WHO, 2010.

[12] WHO. *Coverage of selected health services for HIV/AIDS prevention and care in less developed countries in 2001.* Geneva: WHO, 2002.

[13] The Partnership for Maternal, Newborn & Child Health. *Opportunities for Africa's newborns.* Geneva: WHO, no date.

[14] Wortley PM, Lindegren ML, Fleming PL. Successful implementation of perinatal HIV prevention guidelines. MMWR Recomm Rep 2001; 50 (RR06): 17-28.

[15] Phanuphak N, Phanuphak P. History of the prevention of mother-to-child transmission of HIV in Thailand. *J Virus Eradication* 2016; 2: 107-109.

[16] Centers for Disease Control and Prevention. *HIV/AIDS surveillance report* 2001; 13 (2).

[17] Mann J, Gostin L, Gruskin S. et al. Health and Human Rights. Health Hum Rights 1994; 1: 6-23.

[18] De Cock KM, Mbori-Ngacha D, Marum E. Shadow on the continent: public health and HIV/AIDS in Africa in the 21st century. *Lancet* 2002; 360: 67-71.

[19] Baggaley R, Hensen B, Ajose O, et al. From caution to urgency: the evolution of HIV testing and counselling in Africa. *Bull World Health Organ* 2012; 90: 652-658.

[20] WHO, UNAIDS. UNAIDS/WHO policy statement on HIV testing. Geneva: WHO, 2004.

[21] WHO, UNAIDS. Guidance on provider-initiated HIV testing and counselling health facilities. Geneva: WHO, 2007.

[22] WHO. *Guidance on couples HIV testing and counselling including antiretroviral therapy for treatment and prevention in serdiscordant couples.* Geneva: WHO, 2012.

[23] WHO. *Guidelines on HIV self-testing and partner notification: supplement to consolidated guidelines on HIV testing services.* Geneva: WHO, 2016.

[24] Lasry A, Medley A, Behel S, et al. Scaling up testing for human immunodeficiency virus infection among contacts of index patients -- 20 Countries, 2016–2018. *MMWR Morb Mort Wkly Rep* 2019; 68: 474-477.

25 Pettifor A, Lippman SA, Kimaru L, et al. HIV self-testing among young women in rural South Africa: A randomized controlled trial comparing clinic-based HIV testing to the choice of either clinic testing or HIV self-testing with secondary distribution to peers and partner. *EClinicalMedicine* 2020; 100327.

26 WHO. *Antiretroviral drugs for treating pregnant women and prevention HIV infection in infants: guidelines on care, treatment and support for women living with HIV/AIDS and their children in resource-constrained settings.* Geneva: WHO, 2004.

27 WHO. Antiretroviral drugs for treating pregnant women and preventing HIV infection in infants: towards universal access: recommendations for a public health approach. – 2006 version. Geneva: WHO, 2006.

28 WHO. Programmatic update: Use of antiretroviral drugs for treating pregnant women and prevention HIV in infants: executive summary. Geneva: WHO, 2012.

29 Farmer P, Leandre F, Mukherjee JS. Community-based approaches to HIV treatment in resource-poor settings. Lancet 2001; 358: 404-409.

30 McNeil DG Jr. Indian company offers to supply AIDS drugs at low cost in Africa. *New York Times* 7 February 2001.

31 WHO, UNAIDS. *Treatment 3 million by 2005: making it happen: the WHO strategy.* Geneva: WHO, 2003.

32 UN General Assembly. Political declaration on HIV and AIDS: On the fast track to accelerating the fight against HIV and to ending the AIDS epidemic by 2030. A/RES/70/266. New York: UN, 8 June 2016.

33 WHO, UNAIDS. *New data on male circumcision and HIV prevention: policy and programme implications.* Geneva: WHO, 2007.

34 WHO, UNAIDS. *Progress in scale up of male circumcision for HIV prevention in Eastern and Southern Africa: focus on service delivery*, 2011 revised. Geneva: WHO, 2011.

35 WHO. Progress brief: Voluntary medical male circumcision for HIV prevention. Geneva: WHO, July 2018.

36 UNAIDS. *Global AIDS update: communities at the center: defending rights, breaking barriers, reaching people with HIV service.* Geneva: UNAIDS, 2019.

37 Davis SM, Hines JZ, Habel M, et al. Progress in voluntary medical male circumcision for HIV prevention supported by the US President's Emergency Plan for AIDS Relief through 2017: longitudinal and recent cross-sectional programme data. *BMJ Open* 2018; 8:e021835.

[38] Auvert B, Taljaard D, Lagarde E, et al. Randomized controlled intervention trial of male circumcision for reduction of HIV infection risk: the ANRS 1265 trial. *PLoS Med* 2005; 2: 1112-1122.

[39] Gray RH, Kigozi G, Serwadda D, et al. Male circumcision for HIV prevention in men in Rakai, Uganda: a randomized controlled trial. *Lancet* 2007; 369: 657-666.

[40] Bailey RC, Moses S, Parker CB, et al. Male circumcision for HIV prevention in young men in Kisumu, Kenya: a randomised controlled trial. *Lancet* 2007; 369: 643-656.

[41] Wawer M. Trial of male circumcision: HIV, sexually transmitted disease (STD) and behavioral effects men, women and the community. *ClinicalTrials.gov* [internet] 10 August 2007. Available at: https://clinicaltrials.gov/ct2/show/NCT00124878 (accessed 2 May 2018).

[42] Brewer D, Potterat J, Roberts JM, et al. S. Male and Female Circumcision Associated With Prevalent HIV Infection in Virgins and Adolescents in Kenya, Lesotho, and Tanzania. *Ann Epidemology* 2007; 17: 217.e1–217.e12.

[43] Brewer D. Scarification and Male Circumcision Associated with HIV Infection in Mozambican Children and Youth. *WebmedCentral* [internet] 15 September 2011: WMC002206. Available at: http://www.webmedcentral.com/article_view/2206 (accessed 9 May 2018).

[44] Centers for Disease Control and Prevention (CDC). CDC fact sheet: Bangkok Tenofovir Study: PrEP for HIV prevention among people who inject drugs. CDC [internet], July 2013. Available at: https://www.cdc.gov/nchhstp/newsroom/docs/factsheets/archive/prep-idu-factsheet-508.pdf (accessed 19 August 2020).

[45] Choopanya K. et al. Antiretroviral prophylaxis for HIV infection in injecting drug users in Bangkok, Thailand (the Bangkok Tenofovir Study): a randomized, double-blind, placebo-controlled phase 3 trial. *Lancet* 2013; 381: 2083-2090.

[46] WHO. WHO expands recommendation on oral pre-exposure prophylaxis of HIV infection (PrEP). Geneva: WHO; 2015.

[47] Van Damme L, Corneli A, Ahmed K, et al. Preexposure prophylaxis for HIV infection among African women. *N Eng J Med* 2012; 367: 411-422.

[48] Marrazzo JM, Ramjee G, Richardson BA, et al. Tenofovir-based preexposure prophylaxis for HIV infection among African women. *N Eng J Med* 2015; 372: 509-518.

49 Namey E, Agot K, Ahmed K, et al. When and why women might suspend PrEP use according to perceived seasons of risk: implications for PrEP-specific risk-reduction counseling. *Cult Health Sex* 2016; 18: 1081-1091.

50 Kinuthia J, Pintye J, Abuna F, et al. Pre-exposure prophylaxis uptake and early continuation among pregnant and post-partum women within maternal and child health clinics in Kenya: results from an implementation programme. *Lancet HIV* 2020; 7: e38-e48.

51 Wawer MJ, Makumbi F, Kigozi G, et al. Circumcision in HIV-infected men and its effect on HIV transmission to female partners in Rakai, Uganda: a randomised controlled trial. *Lancet* 2009; 374: 229-237.

52 ICAP. *Swaziland HIV incidence measurement survey 2 (SHIMS2) 2016-2017: Final Report.* New York (NY): ICAP, Columbia University, 2019.

53 ICAP. *Lesotho population-based HIV impact assessment (LePHIA) 2016-2017: Final report.* New York (NY): ICAP, Columbia University, 2019.

54 Statistics Botswana. *Botswana AIDS Impact Survey IV: statistical report 2013.* Gaborone: Statistics Botswana, 2016.

55 Simbayi LC, Zuma K, Zungu N, et al. *South African National HIV Prevalence, Incidence, Behaviour and Communications Survey 2017.* Cape Town: Human Sciences Research Council; 2019.

56 ICAP. *Zimbabwe Population-based HIV Impact Assessment (ZIMPHIA) 2015-2016: Final Report.* New York (NY): ICAP, Columbia University, 2019.

57 ICF. *Inquérito de Indicadores de Imunização, Malária e HIV/SIDA em Moçambique 2015.* Rockville (MD); ICF, 2018.

58 ICAP. *Namibia Population-based HIV Impact Assessment (NAMPHIA) 2017:* Final Report. New York (NY): ICAP, Columba University, 2019.

59 ICAP. *Zambia Population-based HIV Impact Assessment (ZAMPHIA) 2016: Final Report.* New York (NY): ICAP, Columbia University, 2019.

Annex One

HIV/AIDS Epidemics in Africa

HIV in sub-Saharan Africa vs. the rest of the world

HIV epidemics in sub-Saharan Africa compared to epidemics elsewhere infect more people, and especially more women (Figure A1.1). In sub-Saharan Africa, 1.7 women are infected for every HIV-positive man, whereas 0.5 women are infected for every HIV-positive man in the rest of the world.

Figure A1.1: Percentages* of women, men, and adults (aged 15 years and older) who are HIV-positive in the rest of the world, sub-Saharan Africa, South Africa, and Niger, 2019

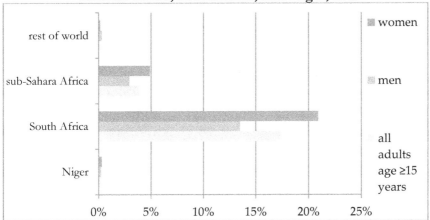

*The percentages of women/men/adults aged 15 years and older who are HIV-positive are: rest of world: 0.16%/0.31%/0.24%; sub-Saharan Africa: 4.9%/2.9%/3.9%; South Africa: 20.9%/13.5%/17.3%; Niger: 0.29%/0.22%/026%.
Sources: Numbers of HIV infections are from UNAIDS.[1] Population data are from the UN[2] (adjusted to agree with WHO's definition of sub-Saharan Africa, as explained in notes to Table A1.1). Percentages of populations aged ≥15 years are from Statistica,[3] except the age breakdown for Niger is from the UN[2] and age and sex breakdowns for South Africa are from Statistics South Africa from the 2011 census.[4]

This difference – more infected women than men – is consistent across mainland sub-Saharan Africa, even in countries where low percentages of the population are infected (see, for example, Niger in Figure A1.1).

The percentage of women aged 15 years and older who are HIV-positive in sub-Saharan Africa is more than 30 times the percentage of women infected in the rest of the world: 4.9% vs. 0.16%. But differences across Africa are even greater: The percentage of women infected in South Africa (20.9%) is 72 times the percentage infected in Niger (0.29%). Comparing South Africa to the rest of the world, the percentage of women aged 15 years and older who are HIV-positive in South Africa is more than 120 times the percentage infected in the rest of the world.

After decades of looking, no one has been able to find any sexual differences (behaviors, other infections, circumcision, etc.) between sub-Saharan Africa and the rest of the world as well as across Africa that could come close to explaining the differences shown in Figure A1.1. (Chapter 6 presents evidence to assess the percentages of HIV infections in sub-Saharan Africa from sex and bloodborne risks.)

Regional concentration of HIV in Africa

As of 2019, South Africa, with 5.6% of the population of sub-Saharan Africa, had 29% of HIV infections in Africa (7.5 million of 25.6 million infections). Taken together, 12 countries in Eastern and Southern Africa – 10 former British colonies along with Mozambique and Namibia, which have been heavily influenced by South Africa – had 29% of Africa's population but 75% of Africa's HIV infections (Table A1.2). Women's lifetime risk for HIV exceeds 50% in several of these countries (see Figure 7.3).

In Western and Central Africa, the percent of adults HIV-positive exceeded 2% in only eight countries (Table A1.1). Together, these eight countries had 7.2% of the population and 5.4% of HIV infections in Africa. All other countries in sub-Saharan Africa had 64% of the population but only 20% of HIV infections.

In Nigeria and Ethiopia, the two countries with the largest populations, 1.3% and 0.9% of adults were infected, respectively. In the Democratic Republic of the Cong (DRC), with the third largest population, only 0.8% of adults were infected; in the mid-1980s, DRC had one of the world's worst HIV/AIDS epidemics.

Table A1.1: Diversity of HIV epidemics in sub-Saharan* Africa, 2019

Region, country	% of adults age 15-49 years HIV-positive	% of sub-Saharan Africa totals (millions)	
		% of population	% of HIV infections
12 countries in Eastern and Southern Africa with ≥4.5% of adults HIV-positive, of which:	4.5%-27.0%	29% (302.1)	75% (19.2)
South Africa	19.0%	5.6%	29%
Botswana, eSwatini, Lesotho	20.7%-27.0%	0.5%	3.6%
Malawi, Mozambique, Namibia, Zambia, Zimbabwe	8.9%-12.8%	8.0%	24%
Uganda, Kenya, Tanzania	4.5%-5.8%	15%	18%
Eight countries in Western and Central African with >2% of adults HIV-positive: Gabon, Cameroon, Central African Republic, Congo, Cote-d'Ivoire, Equatorial Guinea, Guinea-Bissau, Togo	2.2%-7.2%	7.2% (75.3)	5.4% (1.4)
24 remaining countries in sub-Saharan Africa, of which:	<0.1%-2.6%	64% (671.0)	20% (5.0)
Nigeria	1.3%	19%	7.0%
Ethiopia	0.9%	11%	2.6%
DRC	0.8%	8.3%	2.0%
Sub-Saharan Africa	3.9%	100% (1,048.4)	100% (25.6)

Abbreviations: DRC: Democratic Republic of the Congo. *Sub-Saharan Africa combines two WHO regions, Western and Central Africa and Eastern and Southern Africa.
Sources: Numbers and percentages HIV-positive are from UNAIDS.[1] Population of sub-Saharan Africa is from the United Nations (UN), excluding seven countries not included in WHO's two regions for sub-Saharan Africa.[2]

Did something about British colonialism in Eastern and Southern Africa set the stage for ferocious post-colonial HIV/AIDS epidemics? Or is the coincident geographic pattern due entirely to other factors?

During colonial times, people in French and Belgian colonies in Western and Central Africa were subjected to aggressive public health campaigns against sleeping sickness and other diseases, with injections, spinal taps, and other invasive procedures with often painful and sickening results. Did people in former French and Belgian colonies in Africa learn from colonial health care to be wary of blood exposures? There is some evidence: In Cameroon, Chad, Congo, and Gabon, in communities that mobile sleeping sickness teams visited more often vs.

less often during 1921-56, larger percentages of people refused blood tests in national surveys during 1994-2014.[5]

Where more people are aware of bloodborne risks, fewer are infected

In 16 African countries, national surveys during 2003-7 asked adults if they could do anything to avoid getting HIV or AIDS. If they answered "yes," the next question was "What can a person do?" If they said anything about bloodborne risks, the interviewer recorded their answers according to three codes: avoid blood transfusions, avoid injections, and avoid sharing razors/blades. Mentioning risks from razors or blades showed awareness of risks in all skin-piercing procedures, not only injections.[6]

Figure A1.2: Percentages of adults HIV-positive vs. percentages who mentioned sharing razors as a risk

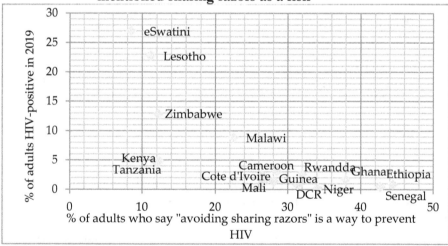

Abbreviations: DRC: Democratic Republic of the Congo.
Sources: Percentages of adults who say "avoiding sharing razors/blades" to prevent HIV are the average percentages for men and women from national surveys.[6]
Percentages of adults HIV-positive are from UNAIDS.[1]

Across the 16 countries, where more people were aware of bloodborne risks, the percentage of adults HIV-positive was lower. In six of 16 countries only 9%-23% of adults said sharing razors was a risk; in those six countries, 4.5%-27.0% of adults were HIV-positive in 2019.

Whereas in the 10 countries where 26%-44% of adults said sharing razors was a risk, only 0.2%-3.1% were infected.

An internet search in 2010 (3-7 years after the surveys reported in Figure A1.2) found evidence of public education programs warning people about bloodborne risks in 13 of the 16 countries. The only three countries without evidence of such programs were eSwatini, Lesotho, and Zimbabwe, the three countries where adults were most likely to be infected.[6]

Because the percentages of women HIV-positive are so different from country-to-country across Africa (Figure A1.1), there must be differences as well in their blood exposures. What are their risks in health care? Do manicures, hair-styling (combs scratching scalp sores), and other cosmetic services contribute as well? The best and quickest way to find out what skin-piercing procedures are infecting women is to investigate unexplained HIV infections.

As HIV spread, people did not see their risks!

During the 1980s and 1990s, WHO and later UNAIDS monitored the percentages of people with HIV in sub-Saharan Africa through "sentinel surveys" of pregnant women at antenatal clinics. Sentinel surveys took blood collected for other tests (such as for syphilis), removed names, and then tested for HIV. Results from these surveys, which were publicly available, gave a good idea about the progress of HIV epidemics in various countries and communities.

For example, the percentage of pregnant women HIV-positive in a clinic in Gaborone, Botswana, increased from 6% in 1990 to 39% in 1998.[7] Because pregnant women attending antenatal care were more likely to be HIV-positive than adults in the general population, sentinel surveys among pregnant women gave a somewhat inflated view of epidemics in communities and countries.

Even if estimates based on pregnant women in antenatal clinics were inflated, high and increasing percentages of pregnant women with HIV showed that ferocious epidemics were developing in many communities. But no one told pregnant women whose blood was tested if they were infected. And because public health messages tied HIV to sexual risks, many people who had gotten HIV from a bloodborne risk – or sexually from a spouse who had gotten HIV from a bloodborne risk – did not think they had any risks, and did not bother to go for tests. Epidemics spread through communities with everyone thinking others were infected, people with "bad" behavior.

For example, repeat surveys during 2003-13 in a large study community in Manicaland, Zimbabwe, found 335 adults aged 15-54 years with new HIV infections; 57% of those with new infections had considered themselves to have no risk to get HIV.[8] In South Africa's 2012 national survey, the 80% of adults who considered themselves to have low risk for HIV had 56% of infections in adults (Table 3.56 in[9]). Similarly, in South Africa's 2017 national survey, the 86% of adults who considered themselves at low risk had 77% of infections (Table 3.60 in[10]).

In South Africa's 2017 survey, the most common reasons people gave for considering themselves at low risk were: being faithful to their partner, trusting their partner, and using condoms.[10] If most adults in the three studies and surveys reported in the previous paragraph had a reasonably accurate self-assessment of their sexual risks, then many if not most of the HIV-positive adults who thought they had no or low risks may well have gotten HIV from bloodborne risks.

New HIV infections peak in 1996-97, AIDS deaths peak in 2004

In 1990-94, AIDS accounted for an estimated 2.0% of deaths across sub-Saharan Africa. AIDS as a cause of death increased to 12.6% in 2000-4. Subsequently, AIDS deaths fell as more HIV-positive people got antiretroviral treatment (ART) and more HIV-positive pregnant women got drugs to prevent mother-to-child transmission (see Figure 7.1). During 2015-19, AIDS accounted for 5.5% of all deaths (Table A1.2).

Estimated annual numbers of new infections in adults and children peaked at 1,970,000 in 1996-97. During 1997-2010, new infections fell 2.0% per year to 1,520,000 in 2010. After 2010, new infections fell 4.9% per year, to 970,000 in 2019. Nevertheless, with more new infections than deaths, the number of HIV-positive people in sub-Saharan Africa increased by an estimated 4.4 million during 2010-19 (Table A1.2).

Table A1.2: Numbers of adults and children HIV-positive, AIDS-related deaths, and AIDS deaths as percentages of all deaths in sub-Saharan Africa, 1990-2019

Year	HIV infections (millions)		AIDS deaths (millions/5 years)		All deaths (millions/5 years)*		AIDS deaths as % of all deaths
	New	All	Years	Deaths	Years	Deaths	
1990	1.46	5.8					
1995	1.96	12.2	1990-94	0.813	1990-95	41.57	2.0%
2000	1.94	17.0	1995-99	4.06	1995-00	46.06	8.8%
2005	1.77	19.0	2000-4	6.14	2000-5	48.89	12.6%
2010	1.52	21.2	2005-9	5.13	2005-10	47.18	10.9%
2015	1.17	23.9	2010-14	3.41	2010-15	44.56	7.7%
2019	0.97	25.6	2015-19	2.41	2015-20	43.98	5.5%

Abbreviation: ART: antiretroviral treatment. *Mid-year to mid-year.
Sources: Numbers of HIV infections and AIDS deaths are from UNAIDS.[1] Numbers of all deaths are from the UN (excluding six countries not in WHO's definition of sub-Saharan Africa).[2]

South Africa: late onset of an intense epidemic

Compared to the rest of sub-Saharan Africa, AIDS infections and deaths in South Africa began later and increased faster. In 1990, only 0.7% of pregnant women tested in antenatal clinics were infected.

Because adults without antiretroviral treatment (ART) live an average of roughly 10 years after infection, the rapid increase in adult infections had less immediate impact on deaths. But even before the end of the decade, the toll was enormous. By 1997, estimated AIDS deaths in adults and children accounted 30% of all deaths from natural causes (excluding deaths from violence and accidents). In 2005, estimated AIDS deaths reached 51% of deaths from natural causes (Figure A1.3), and life expectancy had fallen to 42.8 years.

With the spread of prevention of mother-to-child transmission (PMTCT) and ART (Figure A1.3), AIDS deaths fell from 2005. As of 2017, AIDS accounted for 20% of deaths from natural causes (Figure A1.3), and life expectancy exceeded 57 years.

Figure A1.3: **South Africa: rapid epidemic onset, then life-saving treatments**

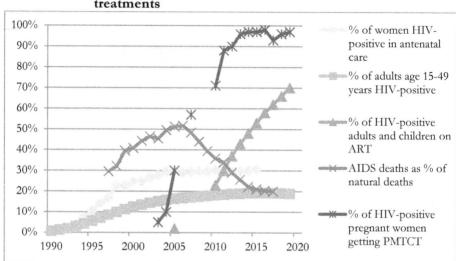

Abbreviations: ART: antiretroviral treatment; PMTCT: prevention of mother-to-child transmission.

Sources: All HIV data are from UNAIDS[1] except: percentage of women HIV-positive in antenatal clinics are from South Africa's National Department of Health;[11] percentages of infected pregnant women getting PMTCT in 2003-4 are from Chigwedere et al.[12] and in 2005 and 2007 are from WHO et al.;[13,14] and percentage of adults and children on ART in 2005 are from WHO and UNAIDS.[15] Numbers of natural deaths are from Statistics South Africa.[16]

Looking to the future

Projecting from current trends, people in sub-Saharan Africa will be living with a heavy HIV/AIDS burden for decades, with tens of millions of people relying on ART to live. Annual numbers of new infections have been falling too slowly to prevent epidemics from continuing into the next generation. During 2010-2019, the number HIV-positive Africans increased by an average of almost half a million per year.

References

[1] UNAIDS. HIV estimates with uncertainty bounds 1990-2019. Geneva: UNAIDS, 2020.

[2] UN, Department of Economic and Social Affairs, Population Division. World Population Prospects 2019. New York: UN, 2019.

[3] Statistica. Proportion of selected age groups of world population in 2019, by region. *Statistica* [internet] 20 September 2019. Available at https://www.statista.com/statistics/265759/world-population-by-age-and-region/#:~:text=As%20of%20mid%2D2019%2C%20about,were%20under%2015%20years%20old.&text=Globally%2C%20about%2026%20percent%20of,over%2065%20years%20of%20age. (assessed 29 June 2020).

[4] Statistics South Africa. *Census 2011: census in brief.* Pretoria: Statistics South Africa, 2012.

[5] Lowes S, Montero E. The legacy of colonial medicine in Central Africa. 25 February 2018 draft. Unpublished, 2018. Available at: https://scholar.harvard.edu/files/emontero/files/lowes_montero_colonialmedicine.pdf (accessed 8 July 2020).

[6] Brewer DD. Knowledge of blood-borne transmission risk is inversely associated with HIV infection in sub-Saharan Africa. *J Infect Dev Ctries* 2011; 5: 182-198.

[7] UNAIDS. Botswana: epidemiological fact sheets on HIV/AIDS and sexually transmitted infections: 2004 update. Geneva: UNAIDS, 2004.

[8] Schaefer R, Thomas R, Nyamukapa C, et al. Accuracy of risk perception in East Zimbabwe 2003-2013. *AIDS Behav* 2019; 23: 2019-2029.

[9] Shisana O, Rehle T, Simbayi LC, et al. *South Africa National HIV prevalence, incidence and behavior survey, 2012.* Cape Town: Human Sciences Research Council, 2014.

[10] Simbayi LC, Zuma K, Zungu N, et al. *South African National HIV Prevalence, Incidence, Behaviour and Communications Survey 2017.* Cape Town: Human Sciences Research Council, 2019.

[11] National Department of Health (NDoH). *National antenatal sentinel HIV & syphilis survey report, 2015.* Pretoria: NDoH, 2017.

[12] Chigwedere P, Seage GR, Gruskin S, et al. Estimating the lost benefits of antiretroviral drug use in South Africa. *J Acquir Immune Defic Syndr* 2008; 49: 410-415.

[13] WHO, UNAIDS, UNICEF. *Towards universal access: scaling up priority HIV/AIDS interventions in the health sector: progress report 2007.* Geneva: WHO, 2010.

[14] WHO, UNAIDS, UNICEF. *Towards universal access: scaling up priority HIV/AIDS interventions in the health sector: progress report 2008.* Geneva: WHO, 2010.

[15] WHO, UNAIDS. *Progress on global access to antiretroviral therapy: a report on "3 by 5" and beyond.* Geneva: WHO, 2006.

[16] Statistics South Africa. *Mortality and causes of death in South Africa: findings from death notification 2017.* Pretoria: Statistics South Africa, 2020.

Annex Two

Unethical HIV Research in Africa

The HIV-related research projects discussed here violate common sense ideas about what is right. They also violate the World Medical Association's Declaration of Helsinki – Ethical Principles for Medical Research Involving Human Subjects, articles 4 and 7: "It is the duty of the physician to promote and safeguard the health, well-being, and rights of patients, including those who are involved in medical research"; and "Medical research is subject to ethical standards that promote and ensure respect for all human subjects and protect their health and rights."[1]

Many organizations that have funded or approved unethical research in sub-Saharan Africa have also influenced responses to HIV epidemics in Africa. The double standard they have demonstrated with respect to research parallels a similar double standard in their responses to HIV from health care in Africa (Chapter 3). Double standards apply to other countries as well. Where governments allow, foreigners have all too often paid for unethical research and unsafe health care that would not be allowed in their home countries. The organizations named here do a lot of good much of the time, but not always.

Sections below discuss selected studies with ethical problems, beginning with the most recent. In these studies, researchers: gave women a drug known to increase their HIV risk; followed people not aware they were HIV-positive to watch them infect spouses and/or children and to watch them get sick and die of AIDS; followed vulnerable women without addressing their priority, which was to find out how they got HIV so other women could protect themselves; and did not investigate evidence a study clinic had infected participants.

The last section lists foreign organizations that funded or approved each project. This annex is by no means an exhaustive account of unethical foreign-funded HIV-related research in Africa.

2015-18: Giving women a drug that increases their HIV risk

Depo-Provera (briefly: Depo) is a drug similar to the hormone progesterone. Women who use it for birth control get Depo injections every three months. In the early 1990s, researchers found evidence that Depo use increased women's risk to get HIV. That finding was subsequently repeated in many later studies. Importantly, women have safe options: many studies have found that birth control pills do not increase women's risk to get HIV.[2,3]

Evidence that Depo use increased women's risk for HIV is important for women in Africa. In most countries where foreign aid is not a factor, the percentage of women using Depo is low or nil.[4] However, across much of Africa, large percentages of women use Depo. For example, as of latest information from 2013-2018, more than 20% of married or partnered women in South Africa, Zambia, Namibia, and Malawi used hormone injections for birth control (mostly Depo, but also some NET-EN,[4] which seems to have less or no impact on women's HIV risk).

Despite mounting evidence Depo use increases women's HIV risk, influential organizations including USAID and the Bill and Melinda Gates Foundation continued to promote Depo in Africa. To challenge the evidence, USAID, the Bill and Melinda Gate Foundation, and others (Table A2.2) arranged and funded the ECHO trial (Evidence for Contraceptive Options and HIV Outcomes).[5] The trial randomly assigned more than 7,000 HIV-negative women in eSwatini, Kenya, South Africa, and Zambia to one of three birth control methods: Depo, an intrauterine device, or a hormone implant. During 2015-18, the ECHO trial followed and retested women to see who got HIV.

The trial was unethical: Before the ECHO trial began to enroll women in December 2015, three reviews of accumulated evidence (from 10-18 studies published during 1993-2014) had estimated Depo use increased women's risk to get HIV by 40% to 50%.[2,3,6,7] Assigning research participants to Depo violated the Declaration of Helsinki's admonition to "promote and safeguard the health, well-being and rights of patients, including those who are involved in medical research."[1]

As for intrauterine devices and implants, the other two contraceptives in the study, there was too little information to say what if any impact they have on women's HIV risk; testing Depo against those methods was meaningless. Hence, the trial was not only unethical, it was pointless. No matter what the trial found about women getting HIV with one or another method, results could not say Depo was safe. As it turned out, HIV risk among all women was high, with almost 4% getting HIV each year, Women taking Depo got HIV a bit faster, at 4.2% per year. Such high rates likely include a lot of infections from bloodborne risks (see Chapter 6).

The ECHO trial had no problem finding people willing to do the dirty work – to implement unethical research – and no problem getting ethical approval. More than 750 people collaborated in ECHO research[5] and multiple committees approved it (see last section in this annex).

2012-16: Following women at high risk to study very new infections

Scientists working on HIV vaccines and cures would like to know what happens during very early HIV infections, in the first several weeks and months after the virus enters the body.[8] To study very early infections, researchers recruited women aged 18-23 years from the Umlazi Township in KwaZulu-Natal, South Africa, where the percentage of women HIV-positive had been seen to "rise from less than 1% at age 15 to 66% at age 23."[9] To see new HIV infections, this location was a good choice. Women in the study got HIV at the rate of 8.2% per year.

Because women in the community were at such high risk to get HIV, they were a vulnerable group, for which the Declaration of Helsinki mandates special protection (article 20): "Medical research with a vulnerable group is only justified if the research is responsive to the health needs or priorities of this group..."[1] Given the very high rate at which young women in the community were getting HIV, the priority was to identify how women in the study got HIV, so women in the community could be warned about what risks to avoid. The study was unethical, ignoring women's priority while taking advantage of their vulnerability (high risk for HIV) to study new infections. (If the study had addressed the priority – how women got HIV – but had also collected information from new infections that might help to develop vaccines and cures, that was arguably ethical.)

The study tested women's blood for HIV virus twice per week. Because virus generally shows up in blood 1-2 weeks after the event that caused the infection, the study was ideally designed to identify specific events that led to infections. The study saw 42 new infections. Most women had one partner, so testing partners at the beginning of the study and new partners during the study was one way not only to protect women in the study but also to see how they got HIV. The study says nothing about tracing and testing partners to see if they were the sources of women's new infections, and has not reported women's sexual events in the 1-3 weeks before virus appeared in their blood.

Considering the very high rate at which women were getting HIV, the study team should have considered blood exposures as well. Did women with new infections have an injection, manicure, or other skin-piercing event 1-3 weeks ago? Aside from injections for birth control, the study does not report anything about skin-piercing events, and there is no indication it asked.

An early report from the study says women who reported injections for birth control (mostly Depo, but also some NET-EN) got HIV at the rate of 12% per year compared to 3.7% for women who reported not using any long-term birth control; "behavioural differences... could not explain this increased risk."[10] Considering that Depo use increases women's HIV risk by 40%-50% only, most new infections in women getting injections for birth control likely came from contaminated injections. But the study does not say if women reported birth control injections 1-3 weeks before showing up with a new infection, or if they reported sex with an HIV-positive man or with any man during that time. That would help to determine if the injections infected women or if Depo use increased their susceptibility to sexual transmission.

Even if women had not been vulnerable, researchers had "a duty" according to article 6 in the Declaration of Helsinki[1] "to make publicly available the results of their research on human subjects and are accountable for the completeness and accuracy of their reports." Not identifying the events that infected women was not only unethical, it was also bad science. Bodies respond differently if HIV enters through a skin-piercing event or through sex. Assuming all women got HIV from sex could lead to a lot of confusion if many or most of their infections came from blood risks.

1989-2007: Following couples unaware one is infected to watch one infect the other

Beginning in 1989 and continuing at least to 2003-7, foreign-funded research projects in Africa tested, followed, and re-tested thousands of adults without routinely telling them the results of their HIV tests. In many such studies, the populations followed included couples in which only one partner was infected. When researchers know someone is at risk to get HIV from an infected spouse but do not tell them, researchers are not doing their duty to protect participants' health. (To be ethical, projects can refuse to enroll people who do not want to know their HIV test results and are unwilling to tell their spouse.)

At least five such projects have reported the numbers of men and women at risk from HIV-positive partners, and how many at-risk spouses got HIV. These five studies (Table A2.1) collectively reported 145 new infections in 723 exposed spouses. Combining data from the five studies, at-risk wives got HIV at the rate of 11.1% per year, while at-risk husbands got HIV at the rate of 8.6% per year. (Some new infections in at-risk partners likely came from sources other than their HIV-positive partners; the same studies reported adults with HIV-negative spouses getting HIV at rates as high as 0.9% per year[16]).

Table A2.1: Five studies that followed HIV-negative adults not aware their spouses were HIV-positive

Country, years, reference	Number of at-risk spouses (HIV-negative with an infected partner)		Number of at-risk spouses getting HIV		Rate at risk spouses got HIV (% per year*)	
	Wives	Husbands	Wives	Husbands	Wives	Husbands
Uganda, 1994-98[11]	228	187	50	40	12.0%	11.6%
Uganda, 1989-97[12]	63	58	22	12	10.5%	5.2%
Tanzania,1991-96[13]	37	41	5	4	8.3%	5.0%
Tanzania, 1991-95[14]	22	21	4	2	10.0%	5.0%
Uganda, 1990-91[15]	44	22	4	2	9.2%	8.7%
Totals and weighted average rates	394	329	85	60	11.1%	8.6%

* These rates are calculated as infections per 100 person-years
Sources: See references for each row.

The percentage of HIV-positive partners knowing they were infected may have exceeded 50% in Rakai, 1994-98, but was much lower in other studies. Based on what has been reported (see below), it seems likely more than three-fifths of HIV-positive partners in the five studies combined did not know they were infected, and even more HIV-negative partners did not know they were at risk. Condom use was low in all studies. Here's what the five studies say about who knew what and how many used condoms.

Uganda, Rakai, 1994-98[11]

The study does not say how many infected and at-risk partners learned their HIV status. However, another study with more than 40% of the same couples reported[17]: "56% of HIV-1-positive partners in these discordant relationships had requested and received HIV counseling, and 25% stated that they had informed their spouses"; but even so, 92.5% "had never used condoms" and only 1.2% "reported consistent use."

Uganda, Masaka, 1989-97[12]

Less than 10% of participants received their test results, "and we do not know whether individuals who come for counseling share their test result with their spouse... none of the HIV-negative adults in discordant marriages reported using a condom."

Tanzania, urban Mwanza, 1991-96[13]

"...HIV test results were only provided if the study participants requested it... [L]ess than 10% of the study participants made use of these services." Among 88 couples with an HIV-positive partner, "No condoms were used by any of the couples."

Tanzania, rural Mwanza, 1991-94[14]

Research participants "were only informed of their HIV status if they accessed a parallel voluntary counseling and testing service. Only a small number of participants pursued this service. At follow-up, only 5% of men reported having ever used a condom."

Uganda, Rakai, 1990-91[15]

"Among the serodiscordant couples, only 10 men (12.7%) and six women (7.2%) requested both counseling and their HIV test results during 1990-91." In couples where one partner was infected, 2.1% of HIV-negative women and 17% of HIV-negative men reported condom use.

Uganda, Rakai, 2003-7[18]

Similar unethical practices continued into the twenty-first century. To find out what effect circumcising HIV-positive men would have on how fast they infected their sex partners, a study in Rakai, Uganda, during 2003-7 recruited intact (uncircumcised) men who were HIV-positive and their HIV-negative wives. After circumcising some men and not others, the study followed wives to see who got HIV (this study was linked to the continuing Rakai community study; see first and last entries in Table A2.1).

Six of the 155 HIV-positive men in the study refused to get the results of their HIV test when they entered the study. The study does not say how many men who knew they were infected warned their wives; however, in another study with many of the same couples, more than 80% of HIV-positive men told their wives.[19] Relative to what researchers had done in previous studies, what was done in this study – following a small number of wives unaware their husbands were infected – could be considered a minor ethical violation. But it was also so unnecessary that it exposes careless disregard for ethical principles. The percentages of men who would not hear their HIV status and who knew but would not tell their wives were so small that even without them the trial almost surely could have recruited enough couples for the study.

2002-6: Not looking to see if men got HIV from research clinics

Researchers in Kenya during 2002-6 recruited men willing to be circumcised, then on a random basis assigned half to an intervention group to be circumcised first and half to a control group to remain intact (uncircumcised) until the end of the study. The study followed and retested men for up to two years.[20]

The study found four men with new HIV infections one month after circumcision. Three of the four reported no sexual activity during the month. When such unexplained infections are recognized during medical research, they are "unanticipated problems" or "adverse events." The Declaration of Helsinki admonishes researchers to report adverse events to oversight committees (article 23).[1] The study's account of adverse events does not include these HIV infections in men a month after circumcisions. There is no indication the study team or committees monitoring the research recognized these unexplained infections as unanticipated problems to be reported and investigated.[21]

To see if the research clinic infected any of the four men, an investigation could have checked when each man was circumcised, tested others attending the clinic on the same days, sequenced HIV from the four men and from anyone else found HIV-positive, and then looked for similar sequences.

1990-2004: Following and not treating adults unaware they are HIV-positive to watch them get sick and die of AIDS

In 1989, researchers in Uganda began a long-term study in 15 villages (later expanded to 25 villages) in Masaka District.[22] During repeat surveys, researchers tested adults for HIV, but did not tell them if they were infected. The study encouraged them to go for HIV tests elsewhere if they wanted to know. Before 2004, "only approximately 10% of the population knew their HIV status."[22]

Beginning in 1990, the Masaka study invited adults found to be HIV-positive along with spouses and some other HIV-negative people into a Natural History Cohort. The study did not tell Cohort members if they were infected. Because the Cohort included HIV-negative adults, no one either in or outside the Cohort would know who was infected.[23]

The study asked people in the Cohort to visit a study clinic every three months for a physical exam. To allow "unbiased reporting of symptoms and signs," the project did not tell staff at the study clinic who was infected.[24] Clinic staff treated Cohort members for "conditions diagnosed using basic laboratory facilities and standard drugs from the WHO essential drug list, which should be available in any health post throughout Africa."[25]

Masaka researchers used the Natural History Cohort to study "survival times, disease progression, and AIDS-defining disorders" in untreated Africans.[24] As late as 2000, median survival time with AIDS for Cohort members was 9.2 months, "similar to the average of 10 months reported in industrialized countries early in the HIV epidemic."[25] For HIV-positive Cohort participants, "[p]rimary prophylactic therapy [to prevent tuberculosis and other opportunistic infections that come with HIV] and antiretroviral regimens have been available since 2004."[26]

Masaka's Natural History Cohort is similar to the Tuskegee Study of Untreated Syphilis in the Negro Male, a widely reviled blight on the US medical community. In the Tuskegee Study, researchers followed African-American men with syphilis from 1932 to 1972, without treating them. Researchers reported results openly in medical journals. In 1964, for example: "The syphilitic group continues to have higher mortality and morbidity than the uninfected controls, with the cardiovascular system most often involved."[27] The US Public Health Service stopped the study in 1972, but only after newspapers brought it to the attention of the non-medical US public. In the Tuskegee Study, doctors followed men with tertiary syphilis, who were not at risk to infect others, whereas in Masaka and elsewhere in Africa researchers not only watched people who did not know they had HIV sicken and die, but also watched them infect spouses and children.

1997-2000: Watching mothers unaware they were HIV-positive infect breastfeeding babies

During 1997–2000, the Zimbabwe Vitamin A for Mothers and Babies (ZVITAMBO) study enrolled 14,110 mother-baby pairs within four days after delivery. The study then followed mothers and babies for up to two years, retesting to detect new HIV infections.[28]

Among the 14,110 mothers, 4,495 (32%) were HIV-positive at delivery. "Mothers could learn their [HIV test] results at any time during the study..., but they were not required to do so."[29] Only 7.2% of mothers asked for their HIV test results by three months after delivery. HIV-positive mothers were less likely to ask. Through the end of the project, only 15.5% of all infected and uninfected mothers heard the results of their tests.[29]

If mothers learned they were HIV-positive, the study advised them to breastfeed for six months, then stop.[29] But if mothers did not know, the study did not tell them their child was at risk. Most HIV-positive mothers continued to breastfeed: 97% were breastfeeding at six months, 92% at 12 months, 66% at 18 months, and 19% at two years.[28] From ages 6-18 months, 121 breastfeeding babies of women who were HIV-positive at delivery got HIV.[30]

After six months, shifting babies to formula was a viable option, and no doubt many parents would have done so if they knew their babies were at risk. The families in this study lived in Harare, the capital of one of the richest countries in Africa.

What to make of this?

Rich country governments and other foreign organizations funded the projects discussed in this chapter, and institutional review boards said they were ethical (Table A2.2). Despite common sense, the Declaration of Helsinki, and other guidelines for medical research, unethical research has been all too common in Africa.

Table A2.2: Foreign organizations funding and approving the projects discussed in this annex

What was unethical?	Study countries, Years	Who funded?	Who approved?
Giving women a drug known to increase HIV risk	Eswatini, Kenya, South Africa, Zambia, 2015-18[5]	BMGF; USAID; PEPFAR, Swedish International Development Cooperation Agency; UN Population Fund	WHO; FHI 360; Columbia U
Not finding out how vulnerable women got HIV	South Africa, 2012-16[8]	BMGF; IAVI; NIH; Harvard U; AIDS Healthcare Foundation; Howard Hughes Medical Institute; and others	Massachusetts General Hospital

Table A2.2, continued

What was unethical?	Study countries, years	Who funded?	Who approved?
Watching adults not knowing their spouses were HIV-positive get HIV	Uganda, 2003-07[17][18]	BMGF; NIH	JHU; Western Institutional Review Board
	Uganda, 1994-98[11]	NIH, Rockefeller Foundation; World Bank	Columbia U; JHU; NIH
	Uganda, 1989-97[12]	MRC; ODA	Not reported
	Tanzania, 1991-96[13]	Netherlands Ministry for Development Cooperation	Not reported
	Tanzania, 1991-94[14]	Commission of European Communities; Center for International Migration and Development, Germany; MRC	Not reported
	Uganda, 1990-91[15]	NIH; Rockefeller Foundation; JHU	Not reported
Not investigating to see if the study clinic infected participants	Kenya, 2002-6[20]	NIH; Canadian Institutes for Health Research	NIH; U of Manitoba; Research Triangle Institute; U of Washington
Watching people not knowing they were HIV-positive get sick and die	Uganda, 1990-2004[22,23,25]	MRC; ODA; DfID	LSHTM
Watching mothers not knowing they were HIV-positive infect breastfeeding babies	Zimbabwe, 1997-2000[28]	Canadian International Development Agency; USAID; BMGF; Rockefeller Foundation; BASF	JHU; Montreal General Hospital.

Abbreviations: BASF: Badische Anilin und Soda Fabrik (German chemical company); BMGF: Bill and Melinda Gates Foundation; DfID: UK Department for International Development; IAVI: International AIDS Vaccine Initiative; JHU: Johns Hopkins University; MRC: UK Medical Research Council; LSHTM: London School of Hygiene and Tropical Medicine; NIH: US National Institutes of Health; ODA: UK Overseas Development Administration; PEPFAR: US President's Emergency Fund for AIDS Relief; U: university; UN: United Nations; USAID: United States Agency for International Development; WHO: World Health Organization.
Sources: See references in the second column in each row.

References

[1] World Medical Association (WMA). WMA Declaration of Helsinki – ethical principles for medical research involving human subject, amended October 2013. Ferney-Voltaire, France: WMA, 2013.

[2] Ralph LR, McCoy SI, Shiu K, Padian N. Hormonal contraception use and women's risk of HIV acquisition: a meta-analysis of observational studies. Lancet Infect Dis 2015; 15: 181-89

[3] Morrison CS. Chen P-L. Kwok C, et al. Hormonal contraception and the risk of HIV acquisition: an individual participant meta-analysis. *PLoS Med* 2015; 12: e1001778.

[4] UN, Department of Economic and Social Affairs, Population Division. World Contraceptive Use 2020. POP/DB/CP/Rev2020. New York: UN, 2020.

[5] Evidence for Contraceptive Options and HIV Outcomes (ECHO) Trial Consortium. HIV incidence among women using intramuscular depot medroxyprogesterone acetate, a copper intrauterine device, or a levonorgestrel implant for contraception: a randomised, multicentre, open-label trial. *Lancet* 2019; 394: 303-313.

[6] Brind J, Condly SJ, Mosher SW, et al. Risk of HIV infection in depo-medroxyprogesterone acetate (DMPA) users: a systematic review and meta-analysis. *Issues in Law and Medicine* 2015; 30: 129-138.

[7] Depo-Provera and HIV. Population Research Institute [internet], 1 January 2019. Available at: https://www.pop.org/depo-provera-and-hiv/ (accessed 6 March 2018).

[8] Dong KL, Moodley A, Kwon DS, et al. Detection and treatment of Fiebig stage 1 HIV-1 infection in young at-risk women in South Africa: a prospective cohort study. *Lancet HIV* 2018; 5: e35-e44.

[9] Fresh. Ragon Institute of MHG, MIT and Harvard [internet], 2020. Available at; https://www.ragoninstitute.org/international/fresh/#:~:text=The%20FRESH%20study%20(Females%20Rising,they%20are%20infected%20with%20HIV (accessed 7 July 2020).

[10] Byrne EH, Anahtar MN, Coneh KE, et al. Association between injectable progestin-only contraceptives and HIV acquisition and HIV target cell frequency in the female genital tract in South African women: a prospective cohort study. *Lancet Infect Dis* 2016; 16: 441-448.

[11] Quinn TC, Wawer MJ, Sewankambo N, et al. Viral load and heterosexual transmission of human immunodeficiency virus type 1. *N Engl J Med* 2000; 342: 921-929.

[12] Carpenter LM, Kamali A, Ruberantwari A, et al. Rates of HIV-1 transmission within marriage in rural Uganda in relation to the HIV sero-status of the partners. *AIDS* 1999; 13: 1083-1089.

[13] Senkoro KP, Boerma JT, Klokke AH, et al. HIV incidence and HIV-associated mortality in a cohort of factory workers and their spouses in Tanzania, 1991 through 1996. *J Acquir Immune Defic Syndr* 2000; 23: 194-202.

[14] Hugonnet S, Mosha F, Todd J, et al. Incidence of HIV infection in stable sexual partnerships: a retrospective cohort study of 1802 couples in Mwanza Region, Tanzania. *J Acquir Immune Defic Syndr* 2002; 30: 73-80.

[15] Serwadda D, Gray RH, Wawer MJ, et al. The social dynamics of HIV transmission as reflected through discordant couples in rural Uganda. *AIDS* 1995; 9: 745-750.

[16] Wawer MJ, Sewankambo NK, Serwadda D, et al. Control of sexually transmitted diseases for AIDS prevention in Uganda: a randomized controlled trial. *Lancet* 1999; 353: 525-535.

[17] Gray RH, Wawer MJ, Brookmeyer R, et al. Probability of HIV-1 transmission per coital act in monogamous, heterosexual, HIV-1 discordant couples in Rakai, Uganda. *Lancet* 2001; 357: 1149-1153.

[18] Wawer MJ, Makumbi F, Kigozi G, et al. Circumcision in HIV-infected men and its effect on HIV transmission to female partners in Rakai, Uganda: a randomized controlled trial. *Lancet* 2009; 374: 229-237.

[19] Kairania RM, Gray RH, Kiwanuka N, et al. Disclosure of HIV results among discordant couples in Rakai, - Uganda: A facilitated couple counselling approach. *AIDS Care* 2010; 22: 1041-1051.

[20] Bailey RC, Moses S, Parker CB, et al. Male circumcision for HIV prevention in young men in Kisumu, Kenya: a randomised controlled trial. *Lancet* 2007; 369: 643-656.

[21] Gisselquist D. HIV infections as unanticipated problems during medical research in Africa. *Account Research* 2009; 16: 199-217.

[22] Biraro S, Morison LA, Nakiyingi-Miiro J, et al. The role of vertical transmission and health care-related factors in HIV infection of

children: a community study in rural Uganda. *J Acquir Immune Defic Syndr* 2007; 44: 222-228.

[23] Morgan D, Malamba SS, Maude GH, et al. An HIV-1 natural history cohort and survival times in rural Uganda. *AIDS* 1997; 11: 633-640.

[24] Morgan D, Maude GH, Malamba SS, et al. HIV-1 disease progression and AIDS-defining disorders in rural Uganda. *Lancet* 1997; 350: 245-250.

[25] Morgan D, Mahe C, Mayanja B, et al. HIV-1 infection in rural Africa: is there a difference in median time to AIDS and survival compared with that in industrialized countries? *AIDS* 2002;16: 597-603.

[26] Whitworth JA, Birao S, Shafer LA, et al. HIV incidence and recent injections among adults in rural southwestern Uganda. *AIDS* 2007; 21: 1056-1058.

[27] Rockwell DH, Moore MB. The Tuskegee study of untreated syphilis. *Arch Int Med* 1964; 114: 792–798.

[28] Humphrey JH, Iliff PJ, Marinda ET, et al. Effects of a single large dose of vitamin A, given during the postpartum period to HIV-positive women and their infants, on child HIV infection, HIV-free survival, and mortality. *J Infect Dis* 2006; 193: 860–871.

[29] Piwoz EG, Iliff PJ, Tavengwa N, et al. An education and counseling program for preventing breast-feeding-associated HIV transmission in Zimbabwe: design and impact on maternal knowledge and behavior. *J Nutr* 2005; 135: 950-955.

[30] Iliff PJ, Piwoz EG, Tavengwa NV, et al. Early exclusive breastfeeding reduces the risk of postnatal NIV-1 transmission and increases HIV-free survival. *AIDS* 2005; 19: 699-708.

Index

A

antiretroviral treatment (ART)
    delayed for years, 102
    Partners in Health provides ART in Haiti, 106
    rapid expansion, 106

B

blood plasma, 23, 24, 28
booklet on HIV for UN employees, 41, 45
Botswana
    Botswana-Harvard AIDS Institute Partnership, 51
    HIV sequencing, 82
    not protecting women, 112
breastfeeding
    child-to-mother HIV transmission, 33, 63
    mothers in research not told they were infected, 138

C

Cambodia, 17
Ceausescu, Nikolae, 26
China, 24
circumcision, 109

D

De Cock, Kevin, 103
Declaration of Helsinki – Ethical Principles for Medical Research, 129
Declaration of Lisbon on the Rights of the Patient, 52
Depo-Provera, 130, 132
DRC (Democratic Republic of the Congo)
    unexplained HIV in children, 39

E

Egypt, 13
equipment to sterilize instruments, lack of, 49
eSwatini
    not protecting women, 112
    unexplained HIV in children, 60
    unexplained HIV in virgins, 60
    unexplained HIV in young women, 87

H

HIV sequencing
    finds few sex partners in Botswana, Uganda, 85–87
    outbreak in KwaZulu-Natal, 75
HIV testing
    AIDS exceptionalism, 99
    contact tracing and testing, 84
    couple counseling, 104
    delayed for years, 99
    rapid expansion, 103
    self-testing, 104
HIV transmission efficiency
    HIV survival in syringes, 31
    through bloodborne risks, 30
    through sex, 87–90, 133

I

India, 13, 24
injections
    auto-disable or auto-destruct syringes, 43, 51
    for immunizations, 41–42
    safety engineered syringes, 51
    unsterile, 42
investigations

foreign participation, 15, 17, 31
guidelines for the United Kingdom, 4
guidelines for the US, 4
mismanaged, 32
no-fault, 8

K

Kazakhstan, 20
Kenya
  unexplained HIV in virgins, 60
Kyrgyzstan, 19

L

Lancet, 45
Lesotho
  not protecting women, 112
  unexplained HIV in virgins, 60
  unexplained HIV in young women, 87
Libya, 22

M

Malawi
  unexplained HIV in virgins, 60
Mann, Jonathan, 40, 102
Mexico, 28
Mir, Fatima, 15
Mozambique
  not protecting women, 112
  unexplained HIV in children, 59
  unexplained HIV in virgins, 60

N

Namibia
  not protecting women, 112
  unexplained HIV in virgins, 60
  unexplained HIV in young women, 87

P

Pakistan
  Jalalpur Jattan, 32

Kot Imrana, 16
Ratodero, 14
Piot, Peter, 40
Potterat, John, 93
pre-exposure prophylaxis (PrEP), 110
prevention of mother-to-child transmission (PMTCT)
  delayed for years, 100
  rapid expansion, 104

Q

quack, 13, 15, 16, 18, 29, 32

R

Romania, 26
Russia, 27
Rwanda
  unexplained HIV in children, 39, 40

S

Senate, US, 44
SIGN (Safe Injection Global Network), 43
South Africa
  failure to investigate, 64
  late onset of intense epidemic, 125
  unexplained HIV in children, 60
  unexplained HIV in virgins, 60
  unexplained HIV in young women, 87

T

Tanzania
  unexplained HIV in children, 40
  unexplained HIV in virgins, 60
Tuskegee, 137

U

Uganda
  HIV sequencing, 83
  unexplained HIV in children, 40, 60
  unexplained HIV in virgins, 60
UNAIDS

accepts unsafe injections, 45
booklet on HIV for UN employees,
45
rejects sexual behavior evidence, 80
unexplained HIV
children, 59
pregnant women and new mothers,
61–63
selected studies in Africa, 63
self-declared virgins, 59
students in KwaZulu-Natal, 66
young people in KwaZulu-Natal, 65
young women, 85–87
young women in Mpumalanga, 65
Uzbekistan, 18

W

WHO, 51
2003 meeting on HIV from health
care, 44
accepts unsafe health care, 98
accepts unsafe injections, 45
asserts low HIV risk in health care,
40
booklet on HIV for UN employees,
41
Constitution, 52
discourages outbreak investigations,
42

estimates 90% of HIV from sex, 80
promotes auto-disable syringes, 43
recommends safety-engineered
syringes, 51
rejects sexual behavior evidence, 80
reports unexplained HIV in children
in four countries, 40
says sex explains Africa's epidemics,
79
World Alliance for Patient Safety,
50
World Alliance for Patient Safety, 50

Y

Yamoussoukro declaration, 67

Z

Zaire (Democratic Republic of the
Congo), 39
Zambia
not protecting women, 112
unexplained HIV in children, 40
Zimbabwe
not protecting women, 112
unexplained HIV in children, 60
unexplained HIV in virgins, 60
unexplained HIV in young women,
87

CPSIA information can be obtained
at www.ICGtesting.com
Printed in the USA
BVHW091357291120
594140BV00001B/1

9 781913 976019